Breathing for a Living

Breathing for a Living

A MEMOIR

Laura Rothenberg

New York

Library of Congress Cataloging-in-Publication Data

Rothenberg, Laura
    Breathing for a living : a memoir / Laura Rothenberg.
        p.   cm.
    ISBN 1-4013-0059-6
    1. Rothenberg, Laura, 1981—Health.   2. Rothenberg, Laura,
1981—Diaries.   3. Cystic fibrosis—Patients—United States—
Biography.   I. Title.

RC858.C95R67   2003
362.1'9637'0092—dc21
    [B]   2003042343

Hyperion books are available for special promotions and premiums.
For details contact Hyperion Special Markets, 77 West 66th Street,
11th floor, New York, New York 10023, or call 212-456-0133.

FIRST EDITION

10   9   8   7   6   5   4   3   2   1

For my parents, Mary Sinclair Rothenberg and Dr. Jon Rothenberg, who taught me how to live despite illness. May we all be so lucky.

Acknowledgments

This book is the result of many people's efforts. Thank you to Bob Miller, the president of Hyperion Books, and our common interest in Beach Haven, New Jersey. Thank you to my English teachers at Chapin, Mrs. Wanda Greene, Mrs. Putnam, and Mrs. Rinden, for passing on their writing secrets. Thanks also to my writing professors at Brown, Gale Nelson, who led two of my poetry workshops; and Carol Deboer-Langworthy, without whom I would never have started to write a memoir in the first place. Thank you also to Professor Keach, my advisor, Dean Carol Cohen, Professors Tomasi and Cheit, and Dean Edward Beiser, whose words should always be taken seriously. Thanks also to Sue Ellen Thompson, my writing instructor at The New England Young Writers Conference at Breadloaf; David Daniels, my writing instructor at the Bennington July Program; and to Liz Ahl, my writing instructor at the UVA Young Writers Workshop.

Thanks to some of my friends for critiquing or offering input along the way: Lauren Bonner, Kat Forcier, Lucy Boyle, Abby Logan, Will Schutt, EB Kelly, Alex MacCallum, Molly Boyle, Abigail Greenbaum, Allegra LaViola, Dave Olsen, Bryan Doerries,

Rachel Lewis, and the 8 North Staff at Boston Children's Hospital. Thanks to Dr. Burr and Laura Basili for encouraging me to write a book about my transplant experience. Thank you also to those who will help publicize the book: Diane Sawyer, Kristin Adams, Kristine Murphy, Tracy Cochran (who introduced me to Joy), Emily at *Glamour* magazine, NPR, and The Cystic Fibrosis Foundation.

Thanks to Mary Ellen O'Neill for her patience and expert editing advice, Joy Harris for her belief in the book, and Joe Richman for getting my voice heard nationally despite my not always cheery responses to his reminders.

But most important I would like to mention families like the Howards, the O'Keefes, the Provders, the Doerries, the Grants, and numerous others who have supported my family along the way.

Contents

Breathing for a Living

O N E

The Decision

I wake to sleep, and take my waking slow.
I feel my fate in what I cannot fear.
I learn by going where I have to go.
—Theodore Roethke, "The Waking"

JANUARY 2000 ————————————————————

I am having a midlife crisis. Tomorrow I will be nineteen. It sounds melodramatic. But technically I should have had this crisis five years ago—my life expectancy according to average statistics is twenty-eight years.

However, most without cystic fibrosis (also known as CF) have a midlife crisis at age forty and some die at sixty-five, so I imagine it's okay for mine to be a little late. Had I been born ten years earlier, in 1971, I would've had my midlife crisis at age five. How does a kindergartner have a midlife crisis? Friends tell me not to worry, that I should be more optimistic. So, I sit in my dorm room each morning with Irish Breakfast tea in my Coffee Exchange mug, the sky blue carpet scattered with papers, books newly bought from the bookstore, and an unmade bed.

Lately I've been somewhat athletic. This is my third time swimming in the past week and a half—not bad. I've also been doing the bike in the gym, which the doctors have been trying to convince me to do for years. Kat, my roommate, tries to get me to stretch first, but I'm not patient enough. It's cold when toes go in, but once I start my breaststroke, the water's refreshing. I start thinking. Well, I took lessons for a while at the 92nd Street Y. That's where I learned how to do the crawl. Now I get out of breath if I try to do it. Last March I was in the Caribbean and the water was the same aqua color as this, except it didn't smell like chlorine, I couldn't always touch the bottom, and tickling fish surrounded me. I even saw a stingray—scary. One lap down, twenty-nine to go.

I'm a typical college student, if there is such a thing. Except that I won't be able to look back on my life from an old age. The minute I begin to hypothesize about when and where and who—it upsets me. I often imagine scenarios in my head as I fall asleep—my lung collapses, they rush me to the hospital, I have to take a leave of absence from Brown, or I suddenly spike a high fever and I'm coughing up blood. . . . I could go on and on, but it even makes me queasy. I think about death every day. I wrote a poem about my funeral when I was seventeen.

Part of me wants to grow as old as I can, to live, but the other part is worried about living. As I get older it will be worse; walking to the corner will tire me, coughing will never cease, breathing without oxygen will be impossible. I will look like I have CF.

Slowly I will notice and feel the difference more—what happens when I want to have children? I don't want to have twenty god-children and not one of my own. So I look back from now, my midlife point, and evaluate.

Summarizing all that I've done in life is pointless. Instead I will highlight moments, as I highlighted my hair the other week. I was a bossy child, to the point that family friends even had to take orders. My favorite books were, by far, *Curious George Goes to the Hospital* and *Madeline,* not to mention one from a book club we belonged to about a bunny who got an invisible bag for Christmas. My dad recited poetry to me as I was falling asleep during my elementary school years. I never liked to be alone. To this day, he claims it is because of him that I like writing. He insisted on telling my poetry teacher at the UVA Young Writers Workshop this fact before we headed home that summer—it was a long drive during which we stopped to eat lunch in Baltimore. I'd never been before. My dad constantly wants to share what he knows. I am the same.

Twenty laps to go. I'm getting tired, but I think I can stick to my original goal. Rest for a few minutes, watch the girl in the Speedo sprint by effortlessly, spit a few times, and dive deep.

Letter writing started when I went to Camp Nashoba North in Maine for three weeks. I was eleven and in a cabin with girls who were all twelve, except for Beth, who was thirteen. We lip-synched to "Baby Got Back" and everyone was shocked. Even then I got more mail than most kids, and the trend continued the following summer when I returned. At summer camps at Wellesley, Bennington, and UVA it was the same—I was the one who was always writing letters, especially in more recent years with lists of 150 to 200 people to write to in a matter of weeks. When I find a letter in my mailbox at Brown, or when I scour the mail that arrives on our doorstep in New York—much later in the day than it should—and find one, I smile. Others smile across the country, or even across Central Park, when they get my letters, especially since I decorate them with stickers and decorative stamps. Connecting to friends when apart, as I will with my friend Lauren over e-mail while she's away in Asia for four months, is a must for me.

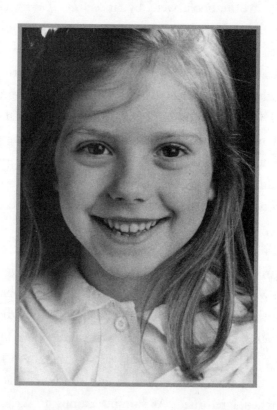

I learned to drive where I learned to ride my bike—the Jersey shore. Beach Haven's familiar main drag is where I biked for years each morning to get cheese and the paper from Rommel's Liquor

store, cold cuts at Beal's (now called Murphy's), and danishes, crois-
sants, maybe even a pie for dinner, from Jack's Bakery. So crowded
in the mornings that sometimes my number would be 40 when
they were only on 25. Now I drive. This tradition, like the one of
seeing how many states' license plates we could find on the island
each year and making a list, or corn on the cob for dinner and
breakfast, was something to look forward to. I only missed one
summer there. I was six, got horribly dehydrated, and had to be
hospitalized—the first time since I was a baby—for three days. My
parents rushed me back to Dr. Smith's 69th Street office and he said
in his nasal voice, *Laura, you look like a prune! I wish I could say the
same for your father.* Humor makes acidic difficulties more basic.

Ten left. At a certain point the laps go faster, I think, because
I get so caught up in thoughts that I forget to keep count, and
then suddenly I've done four instead of two. My mom used to tell
me that *a watched pot never boils.* She's right.

My prom was as I wanted it to be. I nervously asked my friend
Will to go with me on the phone one night in March. I'd been putting it off for weeks. I don't think I even said it at first, just, *So, do
you want to, well, you know?* And of course he was confused. He
arrived at EB's house late. All the dates were wearing tuxedos and
had bought corsages. I was worried he wouldn't bring one because
I hadn't reminded him. In he walked, smelling like a cigarette, in
his tie and jacket with the biggest corsage of the night—a rose with
heather. It matched my pale purple strapless gown perfectly. The
prom itself was not what was special. In all actuality it was small,
since my graduating class of forty was all girls and not even everyone came or brought a date, and composed of a mediocre dinner,
and dancing, which is not exactly my thing.

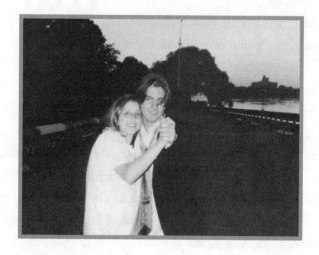

We arrived at Cynthia's after-party in a cab. The rest of the evening consisted of dancing in her living room, having a bit too much to drink, talking on her patio, hearing stern voices yell from adjacent windows that we should *Shut up!* and taking walks with Will. Yes, I talked about death on my prom night, and he fell asleep leaning against a stoop, with me leaning on him. The sunrise may seem corny to others, but it being my first all-nighter, it was a must. I stumbled with Will's help to the East River promenade—across from which I'd gone to school for thirteen long years. Eventually we were all there—sitting on benches, lying on a broken box if you were EB, Cynthia, and Susan, or dancing together like me and Will.

Two more laps to go now and then I will pull myself out of the pool and sit in the sauna to dry off, gossip with Kat, and think some more. Sweat is cleansing.

So, back to my crisis . . . here I am, at college, and I can't write about the future. I can't even make one up because I fear I will jinx myself. Kate had to have a lung transplant when she was nineteen, Marcy had to take a year off, Elizabeth Fleuren died a few months before graduation from some small college in North Carolina. At the funeral her mother told me that I have to be the survivor for all my friends who did not make it. I felt pressured, although I know she didn't mean to put any on me. Do I really want to be the only one left?

I'm on my way back to the dorm now—jeans, fuzzy Patagonia jacket, hat to keep my wet hair protected. I made it through my laps—I didn't think at points that I would, but I did. Yup, just the typical college student about to have her birthday away from home for the first time.

AUGUST 11, 2000

I remember before this summer became taxing. This past year I lived like I shouldn't have. I experimented, I dared, I tested. I wished it to go away like I would a cloudy day—something I have no control over, yet I thought that just by wishing, the outcome might change. Those days in Providence where I did practically nothing and didn't worry that I was wasting time because college days should be like that—complete procrastination.

Next door a child screams while blood is drawn. I want to tell him that it isn't so bad, that it'll be over in a few minutes. I want to say that I'm not that sad, that I can accept what's happening to my body. And in some ways that's true. After the last year I am ready.

But there are still globs of green gunk in my lungs, still arthritic knees, still low-density bones, still a pancreas that doesn't work. Now there's another part of the pancreas that doesn't work. And I will be here for years—getting tuned up like the car in the shop. Except I won't be able just to trade in for a new one when I get too worn out. Keep coming in to get holes and leaks patched. And I tell myself it's not a big deal—it's just what I have to do.

And sticking myself with insulin is not that big a deal—it's just what I have to do. So many people in this world take shots for diabetes. I mean, they eat, breathe, and sleep regimes and diets. If I keep telling myself that, maybe I'll believe that it won't make a difference. I keep pinching myself when the needle goes in, then the pain will lessen. None of my friends with CF had to do it—before they died, none of them did it. This is what I get for living longer. Instead of a thousand dollars, or a car or at least a shopping spree, maybe some flowers or an award I just get more medical problems.

Dad cried on the phone because he said he doesn't want my life to be any harder. And when he cries I become sad. I'm crying now and the teardrops are bouncing off the oxygen tubing. The hardest part is that I don't know what I want, what I'm trying to live for exactly. Do I want to keep coming in and out of the hospital, slowly watching the decline, for as long as possible? Do I want to get a transplant? The disease's grasp on my life is not going to just ease up or disappear, and I don't know what I should do. Live each moment to its fullest and then what? What do I actually do with my days? I appreciate little things. Well, that's because it's too disappointing to think about all the big things I want but can't have—so I settle for less. That's all it is—not a better way to live, just a consolation.

Two weeks from today I'll be heading back to Brown for sophomore year. And I'm excited. But I'm also scared. I don't want to think about any of this at school—I want a break. Kat is an amazing friend—her e-mail last night just made me smile, about how she's always wanted to inject sharp objects into me. She's a premed friend who can practice on me.

I remember before they all died when I was the young one and I knew I could do it because they did. And now . . . we'll see. I'm doing this alone now. Friends behind me, but no one guiding in front. Maybe I like planning so much because I can't really have a life plan.

Since Marcy's death, almost three weeks now, I have thought about my future a great deal. She had finished college, had a boyfriend, had a job as a middle school English teacher in New Jersey. How can I continue here now that she is not able to lead me? I have known many children with CF over the years, but now most are dead. I often feel guilty.

I hope that living without her here will be easier than I imagine. Marcy knew what she was doing, she trained me to survive, she wanted me to go into the hospital, to take my now needed insulin, to have a lung transplant. She taught me to go on, to bounce back from physical and emotional barriers—I'm not allowed to give it up. I want to say it's only for myself, but my parents, my family, my friends. I'll do my best to fight because I don't want them to experience the pain of loss.

I've been invited by Marcy's mom to speak at her service. I think it'll probably be me, my parents, and Dr. Ores.

AUGUST 17, 2000 ————————————————————————

Eulogy I read at Marissa Fabian's memorial service:

It is fitting that the service is today because I was in the hospital and that is where I spent the most time with Marcy. She would be very proud—I managed to sneak past the security guard! And I'm still wearing my hospital bracelet, see?

I remember a year ago I was in the hospital and I was scheduled for a routine procedure one day, but I was apprehensive, so I found myself awake at 6 A.M. I looked out my window at the sunrise and wrote a letter to Marcy. It would be days before it arrived in New Jersey, but knowing that she would read that letter comforted me. Regardless of how often we saw each other she was present in my life. Thinking about what Marcy would do in a given situation helped me to make my own medical decisions. Having a friend with the same diagnosis can't exactly be put into words, but today I will try.

I remember that Marcy smelled like lotion in the hospital. White musk this last time, a couple of years ago I think it was raspberry from Bath and Body Works. She slept with a long pink body pillow once—it occupied more of the bed than she did. Junk food piles on bedside tables, magazines tossed about, a Monet poster on the wall, bottles of freshly used nail polish half open. She could wash her hair in the sink faster than any other patient. My role model.

I remember April 1994. She and I both waited downstairs to be admitted and it looked like she was moving in for a year. Eventually

I would come to embody this same packing philosophy for the hospital. Then a senior in high school, she had a boyfriend named Suraj, whom Gina and I used to call Syringe, and was going off to college. If she could do it, then so could I. She could drive, she could get through a two-week hospital stay, she could move away from home. I trusted her—she would not lie to me about what my life was going to be like and I was grateful. If she was scared, I knew it. If she was angry, I knew it. She didn't pretend to like CF or that it would get easier as I got older. Instead she acknowledged its presence and fought it. Never sorry for herself, Marcy made me want to tell others about what I went through every day, to celebrate my accomplishments. I started writing poetry, like she did.

I remember we roomed together once. Because we were both on a drug called solumedrol, which has a side effect of moodiness and depression, in addition to others, we played a game called "I Hate It When." We would go on for hours making things up, laughing about what residents were wearing, or a less than intelligent comment a medical student made. Laugh, cough, laugh, cough. A physical therapist couldn't do PT to save his life, but he looked so ridiculous with slicked hair, a scruffy chest, and tight pants that we named him Retro '70s Man and Marcy coughed harder than she ever had before just from laughing. Two weeks in the hospital became a long sleepover.

I remember she sent me cards. Birthdays, get wells, little packages.

"When you feel down and out, just lift up your head and shout, and scream and gripe and WHINE and BITCH!"

Written in perfect purple handwriting, she says,

"Who else can we bitch to if not one another, right? I miss you and hope that things in the real world are going ok. Just remember that it takes time and that I'm here for you whenever you need to talk. Everything will be ok. You are very brave and very special to me so work hard to get back into shape, ok? Bike, Bike, Bike! If you start to get frustrated then cry and if you start to give up, then I'll kill you! Keep your chin up baby! I love you!"

She gave me no option but to follow her advice—if I didn't, she would kill me before the disease ever did.

Another card said, "If God had meant for today to be perfect he would never have invented tomorrow." She called me sweetie.

Today I write to her for the last time.

Dear Marcy,

All those years, it was "us" against this disease. Our team could conquer anything from huge zits that no one else could see and which nurse we would have on a given day to surviving the loss of close friends like Gina. I watched you bounce back from bad infections that even you doubted could be beaten, watched you handle more than just a chronic illness and I was in awe. In the ICU this last time you gave me the third degree about my health, made sure that I was taking care even though you were so sick. I want you to know that I will think of you whenever I listen to the Indigo Girls, whenever I have Boston Market food, whenever I am admitted to room 1023. I will think of you when I have the lung transplant that you didn't and the college graduation that you did.

Thank you for helping me be a teenager, for the encouragement, for doing it all first.

I miss you.

Love always,
Laura

—————————————————

Made it back to 10 South, my floor here at Babies' Hospital yesterday. Not sure why, but this morning I woke up, found that Rose Anne wasn't my nurse, and burst into tears. With the curtains pulled and the fan blowing I sobbed quietly. She's in the bone marrow room today by request. And now I'm just upset about it all. I even had trouble giving myself the insulin shot. I've barely talked to most of my friends this admission—I think they forgot about me. Except Lauren, Rebecca, EB, Alex, and Kat. The rest don't call. And former hospital people don't call either. They have their own lives. They move on.

No wonder I don't want to have a transplant now. Very few people will really be there. I'm going to feel like I've been left behind. The service yesterday was tiring. I didn't feel well. I've been here for two weeks and I still do not feel well. I hope that it's better when I go home. What do I want? Why was I crying this morning? What is it? The problem is that what I really want I will never get. I want freedom. I want not to think about the inevitable. I want to have vacations that don't involve hospitalizations.

AUGUST 19, 2000 ———————————————

Darren's crying. Four-year-old Cambodian boy, barely speaks English. He's had a reaction to the Vancomycin—turned red as sometimes happens. Except, for a boy his age it's a huge deal. They're trying to give Benadryl, some solumedrol, maybe they'll move to epinephrine if those don't work first. But he's just howling, Mommy, Mommy, ow, Mommy. He smiled today when I gave him those colored cranes, carried them with him as he walked back and forth in the hall. Then he rode past me on his IV pole, his mother pushing him. The residents are talking. They're going to have to give the shot subcutaneous, which means in the leg or the arm, just like I do with my insulin. I know he's going to scream. I will take the injection for you, Darren. I want to make him happier.

Rosie's four. She has some kind of cancer. Lill is eleven. She just had a bone marrow transplant. Yelling. Yelling, AHHH. AHHH. AHHH. Hiccuping, yelping, ow, ay ay ay ay. Luisa is only fourteen and she needs a lung transplant. Cody is nine. He just got diagnosed with leukemia. Destiny is four. She went home today. I made them all signs for their rooms. Bright colors, fish, hearts, flowers, planets. What else can I do? There are so many others on the floor, too. Jesse is nine—he has some kind of cancer. Joseph. Julianne—I made her a sign last time. Chelsea. I overheard another parent tell one of the nurses that his son was diagnosed with brain cancer and they're in the ICU. What is my role? What can I do? I make signs. I try to bring a little cheer. Why am I seeing all of this? What am I supposed to do?

April 17, 1997 (previous diary entry)

Turrell Hurse. That was his name, I think he was about ten or so. I knew him and his adoptive mom. They were in the hospital when I was in several times over the last few years. He always used to wave when I passed his room and I'd wave to him. I'm in a world where people around me are dying, and yet, I know no other. He died, but I'm just supposed to say, "Too bad," and keep going. I'm having trouble sleeping because I can't stop thinking about it. I'm going to die. I don't care when, but sometime in the next fifteen years, if that many. That's why I am thinking about the lung transplant list. I'm scared. I don't want to live the next years getting sicker and sicker, going in and out of the hospital all the time. I wish I didn't have a "chronic" illness. I need a break. God, could you please not kill anyone else I know?

Questioning

On a slow descent to the airport I can have a 12-hour
    operation to deter progression.
Forget about impending
Live now, worry later.   Worry later,
Put IT   Separate from biological fact.
in a drawer, lock & never open
Is that an expectation? Really?
     Don't want to graduate late, take time off to breathe.
     Blank words, too busy for a hug. All I want—hugs
no loyal obligation, people who do 'cause I'm slipping away,
    taking a trip.
     Friends: what if these are my last years & you see me once
        for coffee? Garbage
I become . . . a hitchhiker in this young shell of used &
    failing parts.
        College students pass in the fast lane
I just chug along, tires low, wheezing engine.
Easier to curl up in bed & sleep. Perhaps sleeping awakes a
    new life & all effort & initial creation gone & dust forgotten.
    My laugh, a memory.
     My name on a stone or a bench or a wall.
Me living to sustain sleeping & eating & peeing
& staring at the moon in her grey cloud hat.
Much I will never

    is the fact that I'm an inspiration to others' lives enough
        to withstand?
     I am unable to birth children.

Unable to ask friends who've slept before
  'cause there are no role models anymore—
who try death on & call if it's too tight.
Almost twenty-something.
I can have a 12-hour operation to deter disease progression.
    I will

COLUMBIA PRESBYTERIAN
BABIES' AND CHILDREN'S
HOSPITAL OF NEW YORK   ———————————

My parents and I all have "soft pillows." We used to bicker about whose was the softest. I call mine Softee. In addition, I have two European square pillows, Hentyle's half-length body pillow, and several smaller proppers. A quilt Debra gave me on my seventeenth birthday—patchwork flowers, leaves, stems, even grape clusters that stick up—covers the bed. Stare at morning junk TV, eat a bowl of Cheerios—I am comfortable.

As usual, *Laura's Room* is proclaimed on an electric-bed-width-door on 10 South, pictures overwhelm white walls. It was my pre-back-to-college admission in August before returning as a sophomore.

Beepers, phones, rounding residents, heels, terminology. I hear both the on-floor system and Naime simultaneously yelling, "Did someone page GI?" Notes and orders being written in charts—Evelyn shouts, "Who has the keys?" (a reference to the narcotics closet), "Where's Figueroa's chart?" I press the call bell, Naime responds, "How may I help?" "Could you please send in my nurse?" Who will it be? I wait to hear whom he calls. Please not Joy, please not Joy. "Karina to 26, Karina to 26." I can relax now; she's one of my nurse moms. Calls me her baby, even though she has two of her own.

My door is open. I like it open even though in 1026 I am across from the traffic-plagued nurses' station. Hospital rush hours are earlier than the roads—eight in the morning and four in the afternoon. Maybe that year at Brown had given me a confidence I never had before; maybe I was bored and wanted to play.

He walked in. Long white coat over scrubs and clogs. I deconstruct the outfit to figure out his seniority. Long coat—important, but he's in overnight gear, like a resident. Important resident is either a chief resident (but I know them) or a fellow studying in a specialized area of pediatrics. My guess is the latter.

"Excuse me, can I help you?"

Without even a glance he pushes on the foot pedals for the correct temperature and begins to wash his hands.

I said, "Excuse me." He continues to ignore my attention attempt. "Hello?" Now he squeezes the liquid soap dispenser several times.

"Hi, yes, person at the sink, I'm talking to you! Excuse me, are you going to introduce yourself? Aren't you at least going to ask permission to use my sink? My name's Laura. I'm nineteen, I have CF, I go to Brown, this is MY room."

Beginning to finish up. "Hey, excuse me, person at the sink!" This time loud and pissy. He turns and gestures confusedly as if I was actually talking to the reflection I glimpsed in the mirror. "Can I help you with something?" I proceed to ask, as if he had just entered the room. He is silent. "Who are you?"

"I'm Doctor . . ." (don't remember the name).

"What are you?"

Shocked by my blunt questioning: "I am a Cardiology fellow."

"Well, for future reference, on this floor we don't just walk into any patient's room. This is my room!" Dr. Fellow turns around and walks out, faster than I could see his reaction. I retold the story that day over and over, how I valiantly protected my space.

JANUARY 4, 2001 ⎯⎯⎯⎯⎯⎯⎯⎯⎯⎯⎯⎯⎯

This hospitalization is only three days old and I'm already mopey and unmotivated to do anything. I just want to be typing away at my Royce application and I can't. I don't feel like it. The Royce fellowship is a program at Brown that gives grants to students who are interested in doing educational projects. I want to get the fellowship so I can travel to different pediatric hospitals in the country and give lectures about what it's like to have CF and how doctors can better treat chronically ill patients. I'm confused about transplants. When's the right time? What should I do? Whom do I listen to? Is it worth risking my life to live a different life? Or will that be just difficult in other ways? Quality of Life . . . what a subjective and arbitrary standard to choose to live by. Yet, it's what we all do. My head is hot from the steroids and my sugar's high. I'm back on insulin. I need to get used to it since I'll be on it all the time after the transplant—ugh. Today is Marcy's birthday. Life goes on. And in a couple of weeks I'll be out of the hospital and hanging out in the city and then back up to Brown for another semester. Maybe my last complete one for a while. And it will be great. I will learn, I will be busy, I will laugh and tire. And then I'll come back in here again. It's the hospital cycle of life . . . hee hee.

JANUARY 9, 2001 ————————————————

Yesterday was my first breakdown since I got here . . . not too bad—it took a whole week to sink in. The breakdown was emotional, rather than psychological—I guess that's a plus. Suddenly everyone, even my parents, thinks it's a good idea for me to go on the transplant list NOW. I just talked to Luisa Decarvalho online. She's fifteen and waiting for a transplant in New Orleans. Everything she said about it makes sense—you have to do it before you're too sick. Dr. Ores told her it was the right time, so they're doing it. Her parents made the decision for her, so it's a bit different than my situation. Whatever I decide I will live with. All the complications that result, all the lifestyle changes. And I can NEVER turn back. It takes guts to go into something blind with no definite good to come from it. She's where I am— sleeping with oxygen at night, IV antibiotics every so many months. And she's doing it . . . so why can't I? She made it sound SO easy, just as everyone else does. I'm not sure why I'm so skeptical. Maybe because I remember Marcy expressing concerns and telling me about how her friend Megan died only one year after the transplant. But Marcy died, too. And if she'd gotten one she could have lived on for years. Maybe it's time. I need to be strong, physically and emotionally. But I need to be ready. I have to go into this believing that I have no other choice and I'm not sure that I'm quite there yet.

WRITING I DID FOR GENEVIEVE, CHILD LIFE SPECIALIST AT COLUMBIA—TRYING TO COME TO A CONCLUSION—JANUARY 2001 ————

I woke up today.

I woke up and smiled.

I smiled and stared at the budding daffodil plant on top of the TV.

I make decisions every day of my life. We all do. What time I'm getting out of bed, whether I should put my hair up or leave it down, or put a scarf over it because it's just that dirty. Whether I should shower in the morning or wait until the late afternoon. Whether I should have Cheerios or a bagel for breakfast, how much time I should leave to walk from my dorm to class, whether I should spend a day doing schoolwork or just running errands, how important it is to call a certain friend or see a certain movie. Whether I should spend a vacation relaxing at home or get on a plane and fly to the Caribbean. Even deciding to go to the bathroom is a conscious decision, although because it's a result of biological need, one wouldn't ordinarily think of it as such.

But all those decisions are different. They affect what you do with your time in life as opposed to actually having a life to do something with. Getting a transplant means that I could possibly lose my life altogether. I have always said that I would never trade my life for one without CF because of all that CF has given me—relations through the hospital, special dying children and friends I've met, eyes into microcosms that I never would've been privy to at such a young age. My lungs are just as much a part of my life as my glasses or my hands. I am the coughing girl.

The question I need to answer is not so much do I want to have a transplant. I already know that I do not want to die without trying my hardest to live. But rather, I need to decide when I want to have the transplant. Not everyone is fortunate enough to make this decision. Most go on the list way too late and end up waiting for months in bed. Others have the opportunity to make the decision, but choose not to decide, which ultimately decides for them. That's what happened to Marcy. Continually postponing the surgery was her way of saying that she wasn't ready. She saw the transplant as a bad thing, an operation to be done once you've lived your life because she didn't see it as something that would make her life better. If one sees the transplant as an end to the life that you already have it's virtually impossible to convince yourself that you will ever be ready for such a change.

Looking at the transplant as a good thing, a new start at life, if you will, makes it an easy decision. If it goes well, then the rest of my life, however long that may be, will be exciting and fresh. I will be able to do activities I haven't done in years. I will be able to sleep for hours on end without coughing. I will be able to walk without getting out of breath at all, even run. And not doing chest PT or not taking nebulizers won't be a failure on my part because I won't need them. I will have to take pills and pills and pills and I will be fully diabetic, which means shots of insulin and sugar checks, but it will be a completely new regimen, something to spice up the monotony of my current medical routine.

That being said, it is still not easy to reason through this decision. Unlike many others in my life, it's not a matter of positive versus negative outlook. Although I have just mentioned the two different ways to look at the same surgery and I can control how I mentally approach it, I cannot completely control the outcome of the operation. Marcy didn't want to have a transplant because she feared she would reject right away as one-third of the patients transplanted do. If it works, then there's no issue. What I am most fearful of is if the surgery does not work.

Diving into the unknown is scary. I've had CF my whole life. I've come into the hospital regularly for years now, I have a routine. I know when I'm "sick." I know which meds work and which ones don't. I have a family in this hospital. I am a part of the hospital and it is a part of me. Having the transplant means leaving my comfort zone, since Boston Children's Hospital is one of the hospitals that agrees to do transplants on patients with resistant organisms in their lungs. It means a new hospital, new doctors, new nurses, new faces, and new rules. It means living in a new city. It means being taken out of college and left to recuperate while others my age work hard and play hard, drink and be merry. It means admitting that I am not the same despite appearances. Again, though, that is a matter of attitude. I must focus on what really scares me the most—if it doesn't work.

Regardless of how the surgery goes, I am afraid of the appearance changes. I'll be on steroids ALL the time and anti-rejection medications that will make my face round and puffy and I'll probably have extra hair growth. My body might function better on the whole, but I will look like I've been sick. I am worried that I will stick out as looking "weird." I remember one kid when I was growing up whose face was at least the size of a basketball—and I am NOT exaggerating. His name was Robert. I remember that after he left our room Gina and I just looked at each other and couldn't believe how much his face had changed. We were afraid of, as bad as it sounds, how ugly he had become. And of course outside appearances don't matter in the grand scheme of things, but if the point of the surgery is to prolong a good quality of life, that has to include my love life. I certainly don't want to be single for the rest of my life. And if I look like I have a huge hairy coconut head no one will fall in love with me—no one. I already have enough trouble getting guys to like me. I don't need to be super ugly, too.

Also, if my lungs reject I will be no better off than I am now, perhaps in an even worse state, than if I'd waited a little longer to get the transplant done. For some reason, I spent years growing up being paranoid that people thought I wasn't sick, that they thought I was making it up. If anyone said I looked good I took it as an attack. Now I'm worried that I'm doing this too early, that I'm not sick enough and that I could end up living less time with a transplant than without it. Once I have the transplant there is no going back.

Just as I can't change the fact that I have CF, if I have a transplant I can't go back to life before the transplant. If appearances bother me, if I find it harder to go through than I expected, if I'm lonely, if I can't go back to school as early as I hoped to, if I die . . . I can't get back the life that I had. It's one thing if it's a last-ditch effort to have the transplant and you are sure you will die in the near future because then you have nothing to lose. But it's not my time yet. I would live to this summer without a transplant. Sure, it's a question of how I'll live, how many limitations I'll have, but I know I will be alive. If I get a transplant and get sepsis right after, I could die in days. That's it. Over. Finished. No more life. And then all this work over the years with hospitalizations and medicine and fighting it would all be over because I couldn't settle for a little bit of a challenge in life.

I have spent my life fighting, coping, and then accepting. Now I'm being told not to accept, that I should just say my life is so horrible that I would rather not live at all than live like I will have to live eventually. And it's hard for me to say that, to admit that I've been lying to myself over the years. And I'm not sure that it is that bad. I think of kids I've known who have gotten much sicker than I am now and not had transplants. They are dead now. In the end we all die, but it's a matter of how we get there, right? I just talked to Kathleen and she said something interesting. Why let CF beat you up if you can beat it up first? It's true. Why should I wait until CF gets me so sick that I can't fight it anymore? If I go into the transplant stronger I will do better and since I plan to have a transplant regardless it just seems like a waste to wait until the end of the summer.

JANUARY 13, 2001

I woke up yesterday and I decided to have a lung transplant. After all the thinking and talking and agonizing, there it was. And now, it's over. And I was in high spirits earlier today. But it's that time . . . the early evening glow when the sun fades through gray haze to the dull black of night. The room is quiet except for the fan and the foreign tongue of the patient's family next door. I've put in a few calls. Left a number of messages. Spoke to a bunch that said they were too busy. And so I know it's going to be a lonely Saturday night. I'm not sure what it is about Saturdays that always gets me down. I should work on my Royce fellowship application, but then I wonder what the point is since I won't be doing the lectures (probably) this summer anyway.

What worries me the most at this moment, though, is the loneliness. When I go for transplant it will be weeks in the hospital followed by weeks of rest in an apartment, followed by weeks still of quiet activity. My friends won't come to me to stay out late and party. I won't be any fun. I don't want to be the chore on the list of things to do. I don't like being alone. I wish that someone would call and offer to come up. I will be here tonight by myself wondering where my friends are. But they don't wonder what I'm doing. They know I'm here. Fewer hospital visitors have come by this admission. I'm not so sure my reputation here will stick. My name will probably fade, too, just like this time of day. Gradually, hazily, darker and darker.

I wish that someone would fall in love with me. Some handsome man ☺

JANUARY 18, 2001 ————————————————

So, I was supposed to go home yesterday. But on Tuesday I woke up with a fever: 101.2. And my X ray had gotten worse and my white count had gone up to 23,000. Then there was a debate back and forth about what to do about it. Some people thought it was fungal, mainly the younger doctors, and they kept saying that I should be on this potent drug called Amphoteracin. But Dr. Ores and Dr. Prince didn't think so. Instead they just changed my antibiotics. And today I have no fever. That's good.

So, I'll probably go home tomorrow or Saturday. I'm going to have to do home IV for at least a week. And that's annoying. It seems like I can't go back to Brown without doing home IV. I make all this effort to come into the hospital over break and it always overlaps with the start of the semester. I should be used to it. I am, I guess. And it's not a big deal. A little home IV. Only two days between being in the hospital and heading back to school.

But I was thinking about it yesterday. And the thought of all I'm going to have to do when I get back to school is just SO tiring. I mean, once I'm there and going to classes, it won't seem so bad. I just do it. But before, I'm exhausted. Unpacking, walking around campus, shopping classes, buying books, making dinner, going back and forth between Boston and Providence.

Despite the effort that it takes to be at school and the feelings I often have of discouragement, I am still committed to being a student. However, I'm also happy to be on the transplant list. I'm glad that I've made that decision. I think it's the right decision. But I don't want to spend days in Boston getting tests. It's just a reminder, just a measurement of whether or not I'm "sick." We've established that I am, so let's just put my name down, you know? I have a feeling it'll be awhile before I'm on the active list not because I don't want to be, but because I'm just not going to have time to go to Boston and fill out all the insurance paperwork and take all the physical exams required before all parties consider me "active"—which is only another word for "approved" for the transplant. And that sounds ridiculous. I should just make time, right? True, I should. But I'm already planning to put my life on pause to have it done. Even after I'm active, it could easily be months before the surgery happens. All that time just to wait.

I'm apathetic today. I can tell that my mouth is a straight line. I'm just sort of here. It's not good and not horrible, I know I'll go home in the next couple of days. But I'm tired of it. Frustrated. Even when I behave, when I do everything I'm supposed to, well, I'm still here. And after two and a half weeks I'm not convinced that I'm heading back to Brown completely rested.

Each time I come into the hospital I know that I'll leave not feeling "fixed." I will never be "fixed." But there's always an expectation that there will be some discernible difference. And there is. I'm not working as hard to breathe and I don't need to be on oxygen all the time like when I came in. But I want more. I want energy. I want it. I want to know that I'll go back to school and be able to run for miles. I want what I can't have. I will always want what I can't have. So I will leave unsatisfied to a certain extent.

Marcy—Afternoons After Work:
Tuesday, July 17, 2000

Exhausted because she breathes for a living
  Head at bed's foot,
    curled to a fetal position.
Bypap strapped on her face
    a seat belt
    to hold oxygen in,
while trapped carbon dioxide aches her head.
    When I get my transplant . . .
    Hey, it may even be this weekend!
Dirty hair and unpolished nails
    wait—
She can't breathe and eat
    simultaneously.

Thursday, July 19, 2000

A scabbed nose bridge
on a swollen steroid face
Shut window shade lids—
  white slits as proof
    she lives
body straight, lifeless legs together
Suction cup of thick secretion soup on the wall
    (I use them for vases)
A mix I made days earlier is playing *I believe in miracles*
    Constant robot breathing

while phones ring, monitors sound, and heels echo
  Constant robot breathing

Life reduced to a sedated, catheterized, intubated
patient doctors discuss in rounds
But she's a teacher, a poet, my friend
Yet to them—a patient
Catheterized, intubated—my
friend

Waiting for the Transplant

The waiting is the hardest part,
Every day you get one more card
You take it on faith, you take it to the heart
The waiting is the hardest part.
—Tom Petty, "The Waiting"

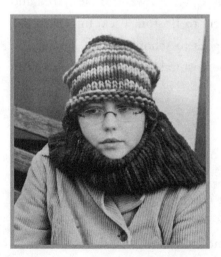

Are you active yet? No.

Are you active yet? No, the 14th.

You active yet? Nope, 28th, pending insurance approval.

Today, right? Hmm . . . no, two more days. I guess it just wasn't meant to happen in February. I've been carrying the beeper with me for practice. I like turning it on, hearing it beep a few times, then vibrating—lots of sexual jokes there.

And then, my ideas for what to do in Boston. Well, I shouldn't have counted on what wasn't really there. It won't work for me to help out at Ms. Holland's school until April 2nd. So now I have to find something else. And I knew it might not, but, well, I believed I could start right away. Frustrating, not being able to plan. And every time I try to, it doesn't work out.

Going active is ironic because when you do actually go on that list you're the exact opposite. I walk a couple of blocks in the cold and I think I'm going to vomit the samosas and pakoras I just ate at Kabob 'n Curry. Indian food and all these meds are not getting along. Everyone's making plans—college majors, spring break, the summer. And all I have are maybes and what ifs. We're taking apart my room. First it was just packing a shirt here or a decorative pencil there. Then I went to New York and we transported stuff from there to Boston. Pack, unpack. Hospital, School, Boston. Stuff goes to school storage, New York, Boston, a separate box for the hospital in Boston. Not much in the big box to New York.

FEBRUARY 28, 2001, 11:48 P.M. ────────

I tried to go to bed, but couldn't. I tried to plan the next part, but couldn't. And now, the more I think and revisit and anticipate the more lonely and exhausting the future becomes.

So much, that I wonder if it's worth it. I mean, I'm not even waiting yet. I'm still waiting for the waiting to begin. This whole month I've been waiting to wait.

Wanting a transplant, but knowing there is no chance I will be called. Yet preparing nonetheless. But now I'm tired of it before the wait's begun. I just have this feeling that it'll be awhile. Nothing is like clockwork. Just doesn't function predictably. I'm not sure where I'm going or what I'm doing beyond tomorrow. In two days it'll all be that much more uncertain. These could be my last months so I have to live it up. Then why am I crying? Live, don't cry. I can't be remembered like this—moody, bitter, unhappy girl who couldn't even get through a semester of college. What a disappointment. What happened? Oh yeah, that was the sick girl. How sad.

It'll be okay. It'll all be okay. That's what I say when being upset about it is counterproductive. Cry and then shake it off. Just cry and shake it off. Try to sleep.

MARCH 7, 2001 ——————————————————

I'm about to go to bed. Tomorrow night I'll be sleeping in Brookline. I'm starting to worry, to second-guess my decision. People have said Brown won't be the same without me. Is it really true? I mean, the bell will still ring, classes will continue, people will be busy. I'm using the oxygen now. Crying. Been emotional tonight ever since Jack and Josh were here. It bothered me the way I was a five-minute stop before their housing meeting. I have a feeling that I won't say good-bye to most of my friends. In fact, I worry that this surgery will become a test for friendship, and that most won't pass. I'm afraid to be alone, that I'll get up there and not know what to do with myself.

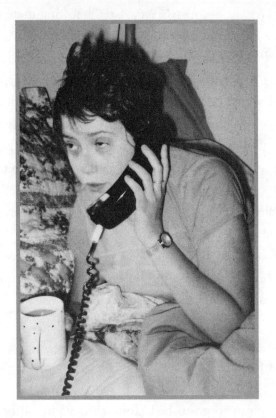

MARCH 21, 2001

Cramps.

Uh-huh. I woke up at 6 A.M. and I swear there was a Tae-Bo class in my lower abdominal region doing a kick punch combination at double-time speed. (For those of you whose roommates did not do the advanced video every day of the week that means doing the step twice as fast.)

Never used to get them, not until the last couple years, really. I didn't get my period until I was fourteen, at the very beginning of ninth grade, and boy was I thrilled. I was one of about five girls left in our class of forty that had yet to enter womanhood. In middle school it was "cool" to get your period once a few had it. By eighth grade everyone was being crossed off the list. And by the summer before ninth grade I was just embarrassed. I wanted it SO badly.

My mother used to tell me how she had extremely bad cramps, so bad in fact that she would vomit and be forced to stay in bed for at least a day. I always considered myself lucky not to follow in her footsteps. After all, I figured that even if I didn't have boobs as big as most Rothenbergs, I wasn't cursed with the paper-flat chest my mother owned before she had a baby.

But now, well, I shouldn't have been so sure. This fall I was out to lunch with friends who came down from Boston to visit me. They even took me to my favorite seafood restaurant in Providence, Hemmenways. I spent the first thirty minutes of the meal going back and forth to the bathroom because even if I couldn't throw up, I needed the security of the toilet bowl. You know how at first it grosses you out when you think of putting your face near it, but then you find yourself squatting on the floor, hands on the seat, ready to aim and fire!

There was a period of time when I went for about eight months without getting it. That was late in ninth grade when I was hospitalized for two back-to-back six-week admissions and my weight plummeted. Part of me felt gypped since I'd just entered this new womanly stage, but even after only a few months I realized that my period was more of a pain than a blessing, and so I decided there were worse things that could happen than not having it for a while.

X-ray techs, however, insisted on pregnancy tests before I had films done because they couldn't possibly believe I wasn't having sex. Yeah, right, me with my dog slippers that had floppy glasses, sure. So, they dipped my urine and if it wasn't tested before I came down the tech would get into an argument from downstairs over the phone with my nurse. My line was, "Listen, unless there is Immaculate Conception, there is no way I am pregnant." For whatever reason, though, I still got nervous when they tested. Maybe I was the next virgin mother. My mom's name is Mary.

Heating pads help, but I don't have one here, so instead I took a bath this morning. A nice, scalding bath. Eventually my body just gets used to the temperature, even though it turns my fair skin splotchy red. Curling up helps. Midol helps, but takes time to start working. And now I'm in bed, my cramps are easing up, as is the gas that accompanies my period. Sheesh. My tummy gurgles and then clouds result. Not much to do. Holding it in makes the cramps worse. It's not like there's anyone else in here to worry about. Like that would make a difference.

Funny. You wouldn't know from what I've just written that I'm sick. You wouldn't know that cramps are the least of my worries. I've been out of school now for almost three weeks with so much to say and so much desire to say it, yet I've been unable to write anything down. And now I write about cramps. How monumental, how touching, how weird. I guess the moral of this story is that even when you're waiting for a double lung transplant and physical pain has been a big part of your life, you still hate cramps.

MARCH 29, 2001
21 CRANES ———————————————————————

That's transplant wait time for three weeks of waiting. In case you're not a math major, one crane is the same as one day. Remember that—I'm not going to say it again.

The weather's getting better now that Susan has left. She's a friend from high school who goes to Colgate and just visited the past weekend—I think she dragged the rain with her. Although Rebecca was here from Atlanta also, and it wasn't warm. Maybe bad is stronger than good. Maybe I'm a bit cynical sometimes. Maybe I just want to blame the weather on someone so I can pretend that I have more control in the world than I actually do.

The sun's out, birds are conversing, and I'm on my balcony. It has to be ironic that I've lived in New York City my whole life, but always on a ground floor, and it's only just now that I've moved to Boston, after twenty years, that I am living on the eighth floor of an apartment building. If not, then I don't know the definition of irony. I don't know everything. In *Reality Bites* Winona Ryder can't define irony. Remember that, too.

I'm wearing my Brown baseball hat. It's, well, brown, with a big white B on the front. Lauren and I got matching hats when she came to visit last fall. Except hers can stand for Bonner, too, because that's her last name. The sun's at eye level right now so without one I have to squint. There are two avocados sitting on the door sill (is that what you call the ledge of a patio door? I mean, it's not a window, but it is a sill) for ripening.

I just finished writing nothing interesting in my journal. Nick Drake is on. There are some kids below on bikes, cars driving along Freeman Street. And a boy in a green wooden rocking chair on the patio diagonally below. His sister's wearing blue sunglasses. He has a truck on his red shirt. Yes, I guess I'm spying on five-year-olds. Right now Brown students are eating dinner at the Ratty (appetizing name for a cafeteria, huh?), maybe off to a lecture or studying in the library. Both places, the sun's getting lower, air colder, goose bumps bigger. Dad's in New York. Gus is sleeping somewhere, or eating fish cat food. Only Fancy Feast for our fat cat.

Tonight my mother and I will watch a *Law & Order* rerun at 7 P.M. on A&E. There's a new episode on at 10 P.M. on NBC, too. And then maybe I'll watch a third episode at 11 P.M. again on A&E. Am I obsessed? Perhaps. But it's sort of like a *Murder She Wrote* or *Perry Mason* or *Matlock* for the decade. I wanted to write '90s but couldn't. What is this, the '00s?

We've got daffodils on the coffee table to support the Cancer Society. And the gumball machine is doing its thing on the dining room table. Garlic is in the wok. Stir-fried chicken and rice for dinner. Avocado and tomato salad with French dressing, just as in high school. But here I can see the sunset.

28 CRANES

Parked on the seventh floor—it's the swan. Each floor in the Children's lot has a different animal assigned to it. I've been on all levels except the second. Logan got in with her mother on the fifth floor; pink sunglasses, two feet high. I compliment her once we've exited the elevator. Mom coaches her to say thank you. I wonder why she's coming to the hospital today.

Pink must be the in color for two-year-olds. There's another girl heading down the main lobby stairs with her mother. She holds on to the mini-banister that runs just under the adult one, wearing a bright pink jumpsuit. She has a patch over one eye.

Stop at registration. Hand over the blue card. Some hospital person told me once that it's like an American Express card—if you're coming to Children's you should never leave home without it. I use that line now. The registration woman says hi to me every time I walk by and then, "How are you feeling today?" Note to self: find out what her name is.

I still don't know the shopping cart lady's name from New York. Monday, Wednesday, and Friday nights she makes her rounds on each pediatric floor reciting the usual, "Shopping Cart! Candies, cookies, soda, magazines, toiletries!" with just a touch of the Bronx at the end. Doreen, a 10 South nurse, told me my first admission to the floor how she once played a trick on some of the kids. She went down the hall pretending to be the shopping cart lady and all of the chronic patients came running out of their rooms with money. When the floor closed down later in the year she was transferred to Labor & Delivery at the Allen Pavilion (one of Columbia's satellite hospitals). She's since gotten married. She was my favorite nurse. The best ones always leave, I guess.

Enough reminiscing. Back to this hospital. Some children have more obvious health concerns, like the baby I saw next door at PFTs (Pulmonary Function Test—a common way of measuring lung capacity). She had cheeks as big as apples, bright red. That's what I'll look like afterward. Hopefully not as out of proportion. There's a brother and sister with CF here for PFTs. I know they have CF because 1) hunched backs, overly thin and coughing; and 2) I overhear a woman talking to them about a study. They'll get paid. Their PFTs have to be over 60%. Well, I'm not eligible.

Sit in windowless room number one. A lot of waiting, a couple rows of knitting. Dr. Waltz comes in and we talk: what meds I'm on, what I'm up to, questions I want answered. He listens to my lungs—a few crackles, but nothing drastic. Still using oxygen every night. With three liters I sleep soundly. My PFTs are up a bit from last time, so I'd been worried they'd decide I didn't need a transplant—after all this. But not so. The resistances, the need for oxygen, the fact that I can't handle school, no weight gain, no reserve to fight infection: all indicators. PFTs will go up and down; doesn't mean much. Dr. Lillehei comes in briefly (he'll be the surgeon) and Anne Gould double checks that I'm doing my physical training—I am. Then I make an appointment for a month and hope instead that I've had surgery by then.

Head home. After all those hours, what do I remember most? What do I take away with me? There's a lung drought. They've done one transplant in Boston in the past two months; usually in that time span they do between ten and twenty. Just my luck. And, there's a number one above me. Better get used to Boston.

Better not anticipate going back to Brown in the fall. Better accept the waiting and try to forget about it. Better cry.

30 CRANES

In Cambridge. Just had dinner at Bertucci's with high school girls. I sit at a black metal table outside Au Bon Pain while they get money at the nearby ATM. It's a busy college Friday night in the square. As usual, Memorial Church's steeple lights up above the freshman yard. A crowd gathers around some band that sings "Baby Would You Drive My Car?" Guys still play chess at the designated stone tables nearby and I watch a little boy with buck teeth pull up a chair to watch the old-timers. Maybe he'll spend his days at these same tables in sixty years. During the day you can pay two dollars to try to beat the self-proclaimed chess master—he smokes a cigar, perhaps for added effect. Planes fly one by one to Logan as people emerge from the Red Line T station and take a couple of minutes to orient themselves.

I feel like a pouty child. No, maybe a bitter forty-year-old who is too old to be young. I can't help but be envious. They are living the college life, flying high at night, sleeping by day. Hiking, singing, drinking, politicking. Maybe even becoming activists, or at least they have friends who are. And then, the boyfriends. They'll graduate from college, go on to grad school, then save the world because they have the smarts and the credentials. Envy. Is it one of the Seven Sins? I'm not sure.

Life goes up and down, down and up, up and down. For everyone. And I don't want any of them to be down, ever. I want them to keep flying, to go abroad junior year, get competitive internships. Wish I could forget about my situation when I'm with my peers, that I could just be with the giddy laughter, brag about living in Brookline. If only I believed it was better.

Thank God, though, for those high school girls who are friends despite sarcastic remarks, and whom I depend on more than I ever could a four-wheel-drive vehicle in the depths of a snowy winter.

MY BEEPER

Leonard. I picked the name from the phone book.

He sits there keeping watch at night like shepherds do in the Bible over a flock. Never dozes.

I know a man named Lenny—funny New Yorker, now an L.A. traitor, who helps out at Dream Street camps over the summer. We started talking because of his accent and his love for the East Coast. He knew what I meant when I said that the bagels at Canyon Ranch were not bagels. Everyone else was from California or the Midwest, a couple southerners.

Leonard.

I flipped through the White Pages and there it was.

It's formal, a tad on the dorky side. Not formal as in debonair, or handsome. He doesn't own anything extravagant, never changes covers, always black. And he stands two and a half inches tall with a MOTOROLA tattoo on his back.

Others have big screens that receive text messages, several buttons, Indiglo lights, but not puny Leonard. Just two small buttons on the front—one gray, one black, and an old-fashioned light that only half lights the screen up. Just enough to see NO PAGES in the movie theater when I get antsy and check for lack of something else to do.

Each morning I roll over and push his gray button with an imprinted arrow—NO PAGES. That means what I expected. I didn't miss the big call in the middle of the night, there is no donor yet. Take the oxygen off, put my glasses on, get out of bed, go pee.

32 CRANES

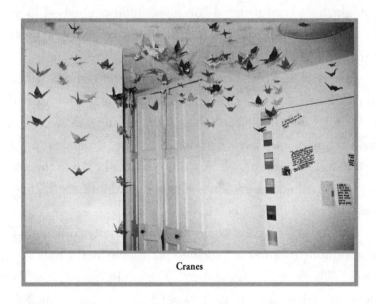

Cranes

"Part of living is waiting. It's not wasted time, you're smart. You can create things in your mind, think about people, about life. Life has moments of movement and moments of stop in movement," says my mother in an effort to console her daughter.

"I don't have anything to do. I want something to do," the make-believe first-grader sobs. "Well," my mother begins, "you could read."

"No."

"You could wash the dishes, do the laundry, watch a movie."

"I'm sick of watching movies."

"What about drawing?"

"No."

Was it simpler when I was younger? Not much. Although it might have been if they'd conceived another child—I longed for a sibling to call my own, one I could play with whenever I demanded, or so I envisioned.

And now, after a weekend of well-wishers and a smoked salmon Easter brunch, I'm back to whimpering. How pathetic. It's spring, I should rejoice. College semesters are only weeks from the finish line. Yeah, well, I'm not in college, remember? So, it's time to feel sorry for myself. Anyone who thinks I'm in this waiting room without hours I'm not proud of thinks too highly of me. Better stop reading before I disappoint.

Just starting to get a cold. The phlegm tastes different, the cough's more irritating and soreness is creeping up the back of the throat. Whenever I swallow there's a painful consequence. Then I have to swallow again to make sure I really felt something. I did. If I am offered lungs and can't get them because of this cold there will be a lot more crying, probably even some cursing.

This afternoon my parents and I went to a gardening store in Cambridge. First we stopped at our nearby Star Market, the only supermarket open on this non-universal holiday, to get some groceries. Then we found the outdoor nursery that I pass on Memorial Drive whenever I head to Harvard Square. Each time I tell myself to drag my parents there. Today I crossed it off the mental checklist.

We purchased pansies, geraniums, and begonias, some plastic pots and dirt. Actually, I think gardeners call it potting soil, but us New York novice cultivators are more vulgar. I don't think we feel like we've yet earned the privilege of using the expert lingo.

Mom and I transferred the plants into pots after a snack of pretzels and focaccia dipped in baba ganouj. My hands were covered in dirt—it even got in my nails! That grainy brown stuff felt natural. And the smell reminded me of Molly's house in Palisades. I helped in the garden there a few times. They always lined their walkway with pansies.

Our plants sit along the back wall of the balcony. It is hoped that they are strong enough to survive that eighth-floor gust. If so, we'll invest in more. Oh, and I have to water them. Is it true that if you can't take care of a plant you shouldn't have children? Or is it a dog that you're supposed to try caring for first? Plants don't poop, so it must be dogs.

34 CRANES

Crying. Crying. Crying. My temp is 100. My eyes are aching. Now I'm sitting at Zathmary's Specialty Food Marketplace having a contraband Coke and eating half a pound of prosciutto with a fork. I will forever be a walking vegetarian nightmare.

Yesterday was picturesque Patriot's Day—a holiday in Massachusetts (and Rhode Island because they're sort of like the wannabe Mass.). My mother and I got sandwiches here at Zathmary's (she had grilled eggplant and I had prosciutto—can you tell I'm in a bit of a phase?). We took them down a few blocks closer to St. Paul Street and found a spot next to the inbound T and other marathon-goers. A boy and his grandmother sat against the tree to our right, a group of old-timers on our left. They had a list from the *Globe* of all the names for the runners, so when a number was on its way they scoured the list and started wishing the person well by name. It was a whole production. Beach chairs, snacks, and a radio to keep track of both the marathon and the Red Sox game results. Across the street from us, the Mile #24 water station and all its team spirit.

First came the wheelchairs, then the lead men, followed by the lead woman what seemed like days later. I started yelling "YEAH, WOMEN." It must be the all-girls education in me. I got into it, cheering for named T-shirts, Children's Hospital runners, CF team members, Dana Farber and Brown. Three and a half hours later we left. And I dug into bed. I would venture to say I was more tired than the runners, but maybe that's not true.

Today's been lonely. I picked up the phone mid-cry fest. Talked to Genevieve, Julie. Called friends at Brown and left message after message. If you want phone calls, make some yourself, right? I tried not to, but couldn't help leaving sorry-sounding guilt-trip messages. Anyone paying attention could obviously tell

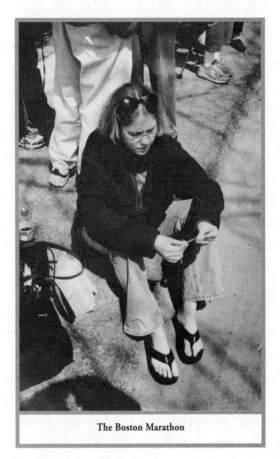

The Boston Marathon

I'd been crying. Someday, when they have lung transplants they'll see how hard it is to wait, how much one phone call could have done. But . . .

51 CRANES

Haven't written in awhile and I'm not sure exactly why. It's been 90 degrees plus the past three days so Boston is in an official heat wave. A nice relief from the cold and yet too soon—what happened to spring? Trees finally in full green shades and flies have arrived. We have one pathetic one trapped in the apartment now. Buzzing is annoying. I started on two oral antibiotics on Monday but my fever has returned. It's not amazing, just 101, but enough to feel slow and leave me with a stinging sensation when I close my eyes for any amount of time. Mother tripped over the cord in my laptop on Tuesday and the battery outlet broke. $278.25 and one day later it's fixed. Ah, those unaccounted-for expenses.

Rachel and I had dim sum at 1 today, definitely not as good as New York. However, in the city I like to go to one of the most expensive places around—Shun Lee Café, so maybe that has something to do with the discrepancy. But I've heard and experienced that even the best dim sum or Chinese or Thai restaurants here just aren't as good as mediocre ones in New York. People should stop saying "quality of life" and say "quality of food" instead because that's what it comes down to. Well, at least in my opinion, even though my appetite has been lacking lately.

Many times I've been told by those that don't understand the disease to just eat more, even scolded. But with CF, sometimes I just can't eat. It's not that I think I'm fat or that I'm trying to lose weight (although I will forever believe that I have a belly disproportionate to the rest of my body) but that when a lung infection is worse I feel full after one bite. Even if I've had a craving for hours, even if I think I'm starving when we order, I can't finish. A few bites and I feel so full that if I eat more—anticipate vomiting. And, I've already gone through my toilet bowl experience, I don't have to relive it on a regular basis.

APRIL 28, 2001 ─────────────────────────────

Dear Number One,

I don't know how old you are, where you grew up, if you have any siblings, what kind of lung problem led you to transplant. But you do have blood type O and you are about my size and you're listed at Mass General Hospital. You've been waiting longer than two years and ten months for lungs. I don't hate you. I'm just envious. I want the next pair to be mine and you're in the way. I make jokes about your dying, or having a fever, or your surgeon taking a vacation. They aren't aimed at you and I don't wish you any harm. But it's easier to put blame on something concrete. So I call you Number One. And you probably don't even think about me, just as I don't think about Number Three. This competition, it's more than graces, it's to live the way we want to, a chance to get back to that schedule we left. You deserve it just as much as I do, even if you are older; even if you have emphysema. It might be nice to meet, to talk about our predicament. And yet you're supposedly the enemy, the one who is in my way. Good luck to you, though. When you do get those lungs I'll be Number One, in that glorious spot that hundreds wish to fill, and there'll be some Number Two, like me, who is not sure what to do.

I received the news via e-mail that I'm now number one as of Monday, April 22nd. Of course it wasn't until Friday that I heard, after I'd been to New York for Thursday night. Didn't even spend 24 hours there, but it was worth the bag checking and airport travel time. The bus exhaust smells different, the drivers are more openly aggressive, the magnolia tree on our corner has already had its peak. No matter how hard I try Boston will never be home to me. And it's not a horrible place to be for a while, but being at 66th Street is definitely home. I'm not trying to belittle Boston, or start a Yankee vs. Red Sox riot (although I do cheer for the former) but just to say that my roots are in Manhattan—they can never be transplanted.

In some respects I already knew this, having spent a year and a half away at college. But I feel it more now because this time is one that should be spent at home. We've tried to transfer such an environment here.

Gus is mad. I think he needs to see a shrink and I have the healing scratches to prove it. He misses me and I won't be living at home for months. Can't blame him. I feel the same way.

One friend on the phone last night dismissed me when I said that he'd been lame about keeping in touch. He said, yeah, yeah, I know, now let's just talk. Well, you know what? Not that simple. It matters that you haven't talked to me for two months. Because I needed you. And others stepped up. Try not to be bitter. Try not to show the hurt. Try to forget.

57 CRANES

I hold Softee up to my face, practically suffocate in her smell. It's me. Some say that she doesn't smell like anything. Others ask how I know what I smell like. I just do. Wherever I am she reminds me of my room in New York, of a trip to Switzerland when I was ten or a hospital admission when I kept throwing up. My mother uses Liberty of London fabrics to make her pillowcases. Maybe it's my mother I smell, just like her clothes carry her scent; when away I used to sleep with one of her shirts.

Stare at the soap dispenser in room 1046. Small oddly shaped room, with a door wide enough to fit an electric bed through it and prevent a patient from escaping. Lately I can just sit and stare. I feel as if I should do something. A friend asks what I do all day. Watch movies, basically, or TV. Talk on the phone and check my e-mail—I'm too lazy to even write one. And I wonder if this is what my life has come to—sitting, eating, peeing. Just as I feared. I'm not dying yet, and I feel strongly that I won't die as a result of this transplant, but life as I knew it has died, in that I have no control. Everything has become about the waiting, it has taken me over. Can't make small talk, don't even feel like calling well-wishers back—what do I have to say?

And all those CF walk contributions. I haven't written even one thank you note, something I pride myself on doing each year. And the contributors deserve notes, I want to send notes. I'm unable to focus.

Sleep with the hope that I will be woken up in the middle of the night, that I will get this transplant before the surgeon and other docs leave for California on the 17th. But in many ways I've given up now. It won't happen before the 17th. That would be too easy. I'm tired.

MAY 4, 2001 ─────────────────────────

For Those Who Are Too Busy

Bought a bud at a garden store
Sat in a pot for months
thriving with water &
sunshine
Until it stops

An expert says
"Needs to be transplanted into a new pot"
Too busy before vacation
so wait
Ask friends to care for her

Two months away
only some who've been asked
check in, water her
Return to disheartened green

Transplant. Miracle Gro.
Watch. Wait. Hope.

62 CRANES, 12 A.M. ─────────────────

I'm watching *Reality Bites* again for some strange reason, we put up Christmas lights and I have IV number three. I think I'll probably go to bed soon. Not much point in staying up late.

I have to stay in the hospital for 10–14 days from the first negative blood culture. They take a few days to grow and Friday's was positive. So I'll be here definitely through next weekend. Seems like an eternity from now and I just don't want to sit in this hospital anymore. Maybe tomorrow they can put in a PICC line (a more permanent IV) and I won't have to keep getting stuck. That's that.

I just wish I had something else besides all of this to talk about. What a bore it's become. My mouth is in a flat line tonight. I'm sad. What am I doing with this life? Sitting here, nothing. Accomplishing nothing. I don't know how much longer I can be juggled. I've been more patient than I could ever have imagined and it's still going. I may not be allowed to go to Brown in the fall—and then what? A whole year a bust. What have I done?

11 A.M.

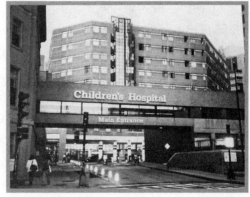

This morning it's just the attending, fellow and resident, Dave Olsen, who put in my IV yesterday. I try to bargain, but realize it's not going to work. Can't get a PICC line until Wednesday because the risk of infection is still too high. Let's hope this IV holds out. I feel myself going down into a state where I just let time go along, stare at the TV. Movie after movie, sometimes shows I don't even want to watch just to say that I'm doing something. I just spent fifteen minutes looking through the playroom's movie list trying to pick exactly the right ones. It's not that long a list, not that many movies for me (it is a children's hospital), yet it occupied me, so I took as much time as possible before it could be called ludicrous. I can be ridiculous, but never the former.

I showered after the docs were here. Put Beach Head in my hair. Brushed my teeth. Moisturized. Changed into a different pajama ensemble. Now I'm going to fold cranes. Listening to my waiting mix. It's the only thing that gets me smiling when I'm by myself.

67 CRANES, DAY 11 IN HOSPITAL, 22 STICKS, 4 IVS, 5 BLOWN VEINS, 1 PICC LINE

I feel like Bridget Jones writing about her life. Except that in addition to having no social life and no love life I am also confined to a hospital. Awake to the distant echo of chest PT and familiar coughing responses. This floor has a high CF population. Brian and Laura Jean are older, he's twenty-six, she's thirty-four. He reminds me of Zeke except instead of a Jersey accent it's a Boston one. He's been coming here for sixteen years and has quirky traits. I watch him soap and Lysol the tub room for fifteen minutes then stand guard outside while it dries. He fans the bathroom with his towel as if that will really work. "I'm very germ conscious." Sophie was like that about germs. Lucy carries Purell. I think it's a waste of time but maybe after the transplant I'll have to be like that. We'll see.

And I saw Estephanie the other day. She and I roomed together in New York. I hadn't laid eyes on her since she was eight: didn't speak English, had long black hair, and was as wide as a pancake. Tiny thing that I never thought would make it to the fifteen-year-old she is now: styled colored hair, womanly figure, tall. She's waiting for lungs, too, although she's further down on the list. Her brother Ricky also has CF. He's probably about ten now.

I've been speaking with Katie a lot. She's having a hard time dealing with the loss of her hair due to leukemia. I listen to myself coach her and say that it's all worth it, that she's so strong and amazing. She tells how her friends are there with her all day and night, how she receives e-mail after e-mail and the phone never stops ringing. I'm jealous of that. My phone has rung once today and it was my father, which doesn't even count. Even my best friends don't realize that one day in here is like weeks. Now that everyone's left school I feel more alone than ever. I'm sure most don't even know I'm in the hospital. You'd think after all my efforts in friendship . . . I wish I could say that people have been amazing. I guess when they've dealt with it nonstop for so many years it gets old. Perhaps I'm being melodramatic, but sometimes I can't help it. I just want to get these lungs and get home. I'm through with waiting. Time to cry.

68 CRANES

Today I lost it and cried the whole time I spoke with Laura, my psychologist. I sounded so bitter and angry and hopeless. But I don't seem to be able to tell my friends the truth. I say that I'm down, but I don't go into the details. I only put the lights on at night when Patty the bitchy head of the floor isn't here. I practically cried talking to a resident earlier. When I tear up in front of them I'm definitely on the edge. My current sob song is "At This Point in My Life," by Tracy Chapman. It's about how life's journey can seem riddled with mistakes when observed from a particular moment. Could anything be more perfect? Julie Falender, Louella, and Mumi all came to visit today. Lauren and her dad were here in the morning, too. But then they leave. I'm watching *Law & Order* reruns my father tapes because there's no cable in the hospital. I need to stop wasting time being upset.

Laura says I need to mourn for all of it now. What I have given up, what I'm currently missing, and what I will have to give up afterward. It's understandable to be upset. And afterward, this wait, day to day, won't seem like it was a big deal. A few months in a lifetime is nothing. But during it, a day is like a year, especially in the hospital. And waiting even two more weeks seems unbearable. I'm losing faith. Gotta hold on, gotta hold on. "Well, darling, hang in there," Ben said before we got off the phone.

Just now I finished yet another Swiss Miss chocolate pudding—my new obsession. Not ice cream, not chunky, just right.

They all knock before entering. Must be another hospital policy. Even if the door's open. Dr. Sheares is the only one in New York who ever knocks. I've commented on it because of its rarity. She says it's your room, I should ask if I can come in. Privacy. Here it seems impersonal, not a thoughtful response but something studied in a manual or programmed into a robot. Nevertheless I prefer knocking.

Just had a conversation with Dave Olsen. He is quiet, a Ph.D., probably smart. Older physicians in training, those with more life experience, are softer, more understanding at times. They thought a little more before med school or at least during it, they're not just about money-making or a title.

The housekeeper here does not sing in the mornings like Carmen does. There are no Filipino night nurses who speak to each other about doctors as the same doctors sit cluelessly in the nurses' station. Like Angie. She does have a temper.

When I was younger she was scary, stern hardened face. But gradually I saw she would bend the rules if you deserved it, she was one of the most competent nurses, she cared enough to stay despite bad nurse managers and shitty schedules. In the last years she did my PT in the night whether she was my nurse or not. If I was coughing, I'd do a neb and the nurse would say I'll get Angie. She works so much overtime she's on practically every night. The loud clapping starts, beating rhythmically like few know how. Wakes others up it's so loud. Coughing worsens, but eventually subsides to force. Fall asleep in a side position. No one believes I can sleep with all that noise. Maybe it's because I grew up in a city on a crosstown street. But I think it's just Angie's touch.

Katie calls. She says she doesn't know what she'd do without me. Most won't understand me for years, I guess, until middle age or a diagnosis I hope none of them get. She's shaving her head. I tell her it will be okay. That it's tough now, but then she'll learn to cope. And then I wonder if I will be able to follow my own advice when it's my body that's changing, my face that doesn't look right anymore, my eyebrows that are bushy and overgrown. I'm not so confident. She says she can't do it. I tell her she can. Well, what if I can't do it? No one answers.

70 CRANES ───────────────────────

Rechelle just called. Impeccable timing. I was sobbing. That deep cry that you choke back, that hurts your abdomen, makes your head ache, dries out your eyes. I awake each morning to the distant sound of chest PT. That faint echo of a cupped slap on the back.

DAY 17 IN HOSPITAL: ON MY WAY OUT, BACK TO THE BOSTON APARTMENT TO WAIT, AFTER COMPLETING THE TREATMENT FOR A FUNGAL INFECTION IN MY LINE ───────

Little Sarah gets her chest PT next door and keeps giggling. She didn't cough once. One day, when she's older and sicker, she won't be able to laugh without going into a coughing fit. I hope that one day soon I will laugh like her.

Last night I met the residents down in the Prouty garden. It was cold, but the air was comforting. Less stuffy than hospital air. I'm on my way out of this new place, and all I want to do is just come back IN. Tonight, tomorrow, sometime soon. Have to finish packing.

MAY 27, 2001 ──────────────────────

I have lost count. Completely. I guess I could go back and figure out what date was a certain number of cranes, but I'm not sure if it's worth it. I have a pile of cranes on the coffee table and I have yet to hang them. Some from the hospital, leftover ones from the common room in the new dorm and a shoe box full that Diana Fishman brought with her today. The last bunch smell like leather.

Although friends have been in and out since my hospital departure, I feel very much that I have nothing to do. They stay a few hours as they pass through town. Jess was headed home to Hanover. Josh, AJ, and Jack were headed to Amherst. Chris and Diana came for a few hours, then back to Providence. Alex came from New York, then took a train down to Providence a few hours later. She's going on a road trip cross-country with several friends from Brown. And in between all the back and forth these busy twenty-year-olds stopped to see me. It helps.

But on Sunday night I'm in the apartment with my mom with nothing planned for Monday. Tuesday I have a psychology appointment. Friday is my monthly sinus irrigation with Dr. Jones. And beyond that, I don't know. There's unpacking to do, birthday presents to find, showers to take, beaches to explore. Maybe the Museum of Fine Arts, the duck tour. Yet I am never in what I do. The focus is gone, the zest is no longer there. I smile to be polite, I answer the phone, when it actually rings, because I should. How did I get here? Moments when I think I should throw in the towel, pack up and go back home. Tried it for a few months and it didn't work. I can't do it, though. The longer you wait, the harder it is to give it up. You keep telling yourself, I've waited this long, how much longer can it really be?

Shouldn't think about it. That's what EVERYONE tells me.

But what else is there? I am unable to live as I would like until the transplant, despite all efforts to avoid such feelings. Alex thought I was happier now. Am I? Used to it. Briefly elated to be out of the hospital, able to drive again.

This Sunday of Memorial Day weekend has been fogged over, almost misty. The white has stayed the same color all day, no change in light. I don't care. I'm not at a barbecue, I don't have a Monday off. In fact, I like the cool air, the rainy atmosphere. Sort of fits my mood.

MAY 28, 2001 ——————————————————————

I've been having a hard time. Harder than ever. Quite depressed. Mainly, just unable to fathom waiting for what could be another month, unable to look at the little things I've been occupying myself with as meaningful for much longer. My psychologist called to tell me tonight that they'd had a call that they had to turn down over the weekend. It's great to know that there's been action, but at this point it doesn't make me feel better. Sorry to sound so melodramatic and down, but I don't see much reason to pretend otherwise. I watched the video from my going-away potluck dinner in March the other night and all these people kept saying how much I live each day to the fullest . . . what bull. It's the opposite of true. I wake up in the mornings and frown because, well, I've woken up without a phone call. Positive thinking, right?

Anyway, friends visited this weekend, but even that seems to be short-lived. My mom and I saw *Shrek* today—pretty funny. Eddie Murphy always makes me laugh.

JUNE 8, 2001

After eight days here, losing 500 ccs of blood, having a pee catheter, a pulmonary embolization, and immense chest pain and nausea that seems to be ongoing, I've made an executive decision to leave tomorrow. Who knows if it will hold any weight, but I did tell the pulmonary fellow in very straight terms that I was not going to sit here if they aren't doing anything interesting with me. I can do IV antibiotics at home. Well, not my real home, but the Brookline apartment. Mom went back to New York today. A week ago she made it all the way to New Haven on the train and then came right back to Boston. Debra took the shuttle from Westchester Airport to Logan. They were both here by the time the four-and-a-half-hour pulmonary embolization procedure was done to stop the bleeding in my lungs.

JUNE 13, 2001 ───────────────────────

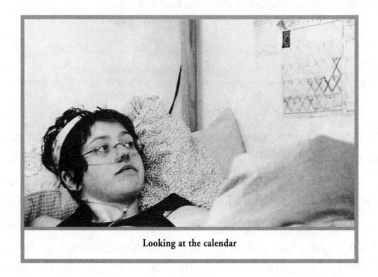

Looking at the calendar

Finished home IV today and got the PICC taken out . . . much nicer NOT having one. Absolutely exhausted and basically the doctors just said, well, you need a transplant and there isn't much to do. They didn't keep me on IVs because it's been a month now and they don't seem to be doing all that much. Everyone is in agreement that I took a hit from the embolization and that the swelling in the lungs and the hematoma by the esophagus will take time to mend. I'm down to 119, a record low for the last couple years and my appetite is not back yet. I hope that my retic count has gone up and I won't have to start some kind of red blood cell injection. BUT, Lauren is here and she and my dad are doing their best to keep me cheerful, get me stuff, and all but force-feeding me. . . . Do you want this? how about this? you're sure you don't want? It's very sweet. I don't know what I'd do without her. And, in general, I've just sort of come to peace with waiting, resigned to take what comes as it comes and I'm just not as angry as I was. There was a call Saturday night, but again it was not a good enough pair.

JUNE 14, 2001 ────────────────────

I wrote this e-mail to Louella, Ben, Ali, Adam, Brooke, and Eric:

hey guys

just wanted to send a quick e-mail to say that I was very happy to see all of you today. Although my visit was not long and your time was scarce I'm glad it worked out. I sat on the main green for a while before leaving by myself. It was quiet. A tour came by. I thought about where I was three years ago taking that tour: that I felt well, that I was excited for college and thought it would be nothing but fun. And although deep down I do feel that many have not lived up to expectations, there are some that I know I am fortunate to have in my corner, that I could never have imagined or envisioned (talent, perseverance, loyalty, CHARACTER) three years ago on the tour. You are all in that category.

L

——————————————————

My energy level has sunk even lower. Basically if it were a child, it would be drowning. And the appetite is the definition of bland. And today I drank an Ensure shake—flashback to sixth and seventh grades. One in the morning, one at night, and fighting about it all day long. We even had a special shake glass—extra big, dark green, fancy. Today I sat in bed drinking the shake being coaxed by Lucy to drink up, prodded to have just one more strawberry and question: What is going on with my body? Why does it feel so different? Why can't I feel okay? No appetite, no energy, just sick. I want my port-a-cath back, I want another g-tube. Just feed me through IV tubes, give me IV antibiotics and knock me out until the fateful call. And if I never wake up it'll be easier than watching myself slowly fade away while others are in Europe and working hard at summer jobs.

Am I dying? I don't know yet. But it's different than it was a month ago. A Cambridge shopping trip exhausts me, when it never used to before. And I'm sure when I'm permanently on oxygen I'll think my current situation is luxurious. But now it isn't.

——————————————————

The sky's tummy is rumbling and crackling tonight. Is there mucus taking up space in his stomach, too? Probably not. But the summer storm is dramatic, how it's so quiet and then suddenly rain and wind to the point that you can't make out the scenery from the window. The bolts shock me. Rebecca makes a joke about getting lungs from someone who was struck by lightning. Chuckle. Three people guessed that the transplant would happen today, including my father. They still have four hours to win the bet.

Back to Fegan 5 and Dr. Waltz's transplant clinic. This basically means that all members of the transplant "team" are available if needed for consultation. Anne Gould, the physical therapist, talks about exercise. Try to keep walking, etc. Sets us up with a chest PT company so that a therapist can come in and do it several times a week. Instead of moaning I actually agree. What happened to Laura? I hate chest PT! But at this point the mucus is too overwhelming. I need more help. At least for a bit.

In he walks, my main man, Dr. Waltz. Oval glasses, children's tie, not that tall, but intelligent. He scribbles notes in illegible handwriting as I tell my story of vomiting mucus and exhaustion. I always make a few jokes with him because I can tell he gets a kick out of it.

"So, I threw up all this mucus. And then I ate some chicken."

Perhaps only funny to doctors and individual patients at specific moments, but it got a laugh. When he examined me I looked at his ID and told him the picture didn't do him justice. Apparently the previous patient, a four-year-old blond, had asked if the man in the picture was him.

"What does that mean?" Laugh.

Then he says what he thinks. First, we should start the Epogen to help my body make more red blood cells. That's an

injection sub-q several times a week. Then, there were decisions
to make.

Option 1: The easiest. Go into the hospital and get IVs and
stuff there.

Option 2: Get a PICC line placed outpatient, do home IV,
take five days of low-dose Prednisone.

Of course, I chose number two. Oh, and I have to drink more
Ensures and eat as much as I can. Try little meals more often.

Luckily Paula, the PICC nurse extraordinare, has agreed to
give it a try after her meeting. Two hours to kill while I wait to
get the PICC placed. Sit in the garden in the shade, right at the
front where all the action is. A large group of twenty-somethings
sits farther away eating lunch—new interns. I decide to go for it
after some coaching from Zucker on the phone.

"Hello. Excuse me, you over there, can you listen please? I'm
sorry to interrupt your lunch but I just wanted to let you know
that my name is Laura, I am twenty years old, I have CF and I'm
waiting for a double lung transplant. So, if you have any questions about internship I am sitting right over there and I'm a
professional patient. It doesn't have to be about CF, it can be
about anything to do with the hospital." Laughing.

"Would you like to join us?" asks the upcoming chief.

"Thank you, but I'm not feeling that well and I'm trying
not to do too much talking, so I'd rather just answer specific
questions."

There was a bit more conversation and then more thank yous
and I went back to my Coke and other belongings. It felt good.
Empowering.

Three other CF patients happen to sit down in front of me

and my mother on the grass and overhear me talking on the phone about CF. One turns his head and says that's what we have. I had already made the diagnosis. Clubbed nails, hunched backs, thin legs, big trays of food, PICC lines, old for a children's hospital—giveaways. One was thirty-three, another twenty-nine, and the youngest nineteen. The oldest was only diagnosed at age twenty-seven! I almost believe his disease shouldn't be called Cystic Fibrosis. CF is about growing up sick, knowing and facing it your whole life, not about being diagnosed as you would cancer or something else. To me that's part of it. Granted, some get diagnosed six months after birth or four years old, but that's pretty much knowing from birth. It's weird. He knows what it means to think you are a totally healthy person, to not have it in the back of your head that you are going to die.

And I don't think before now that I really understood how much separates me and the rest. I think of forty as old; others say it's young. I am living on a day-to-day basis now, while a day to most is a matter of where to meet whomever when, and then how to get there.

I do not have cancer. Both illnesses, completely different. There is no protocol, no predictability, no percentage. I rarely feel that medication is poison; instead I find it useless. And I will never have the realistic hope of being cured. Mine is chronic, like a book that goes on and on. And even within the chronic illness there is a difference from patient to patient. In addition to physical ones, there are the psychosocial, etc., that influence the illness as well. Now I sound like a textbook. I don't mean to. It's just an observation. I feel now as if I'm watching details more intently. It's sort of strange: slowing down my speech and movement.

JUNE 21, 2001 ————————————————

First day of summer . . . hmm . . . Definitely thought I'd have lungs by now a few months ago.

Of course it sucked when I woke up coughing this morning at 5:30. I didn't really get back to sleep until 8:00! Then the nursing company called at 9:15 so the nice rest I might have had was shot.

Oh, well, maybe I'll nap later.

Here's my exciting itinerary for today:

10:30 IV nurse arrives, changes PICC dressing, starts medications

11:00 (starting tomorrow) The chest PT guy comes over

12:00 Trainer arrives—we do stretching and one weight for the left arm (can't lift with the PICC line in the right one)

1:00 My dad arrives from New York . . . probably have lunch, drink an Ensure

5:00 Do more IV antibiotics

Dinner? If I'm hungry, another Ensure shake?

7:00 Lucy is supposed to drop in for a couple hours

11:00 *Law & Order* on A&E

SINKING ————————————————————————————

A June Saturday. The 23rd to be exact.

Lucy and Lauren, both mere twenty-year-old permit holders, are on an illegal trip to Star Market.

Sit on the blue slipcover couch propped on purple velvet. Light changes shade on the wall. Understanding aches throughout; eyes release futile tears.

It is no longer about wanting.

The slow descent to the airport has begun.

It's about needing.

JUNE 24, 2001 ——————————————————————————

There was an article in the Sunday *Times* this morning about living organ donors. Then tonight there's something on the news about a walk for liver disease and raising awareness for liver transplants. In *Airplane,* which I watched yesterday, the sick girl on the airplane is going to have a heart transplant. Today I'm feeling a bit better, whatever. I'm a bit down tonight. It'll pass. Although it seems as if I will be here forever.

JUNE 30, 2001 ——————————————————————————

I sit down on the bed and stub my toe on the stupid IV pole. I mistakenly go to lift up my shirt to flush the port and am once again reminded that the port isn't there anymore. The PICC line

resists when I flush. Start the Cipro. Beeping. Air-in-line. SHUT
UP! Fix it. Now 12 ccs have infused.

At this moment I'm in a no-good-terrible-very-bad-mood,
similar to that of Alexander in the children's book or Oscar the
Grouch's never-ending pessimism. Lightning flash, thunder crash.
I miss New York. Thunder. Didn't win Scrabble. Thunder.

Today we went to the Fenway 13, one of many multiplex
movie theaters in the Boston area. I accidentally poured too much
salt on Noah's popcorn, although the intent was debatable, and
then honestly put too much on mine. The first couple in front of
us began talking about my coughing instantly. Oddly enough, I
barely noticed. But Debra was quite bothered by it. They moved
before the previews even started.

The next couple looked back after a few coughs at which
point Debra leaned over and told them in a polite New York
tone that I was going to cough throughout the movie so if they
had a problem with it they should just move now. Both men
looked at each other, whispered, and decided to stay. Previews
lasted at least fifteen minutes by which point the 12:30 show-
ing was packed.

I didn't even think I'd coughed that much. But when the
credits were rolling, the lights up and the moviegoers exiting, a
man on the other side of the theater yelled, "Thanks for coughing!" Laughter. The realization was delayed. Oh wait, he's talking
about me. But it was too late to find his face among the crowd.
He was a slightly overweight thirty-something or middle-aged
white man. Brown hair. I wish I could've glared. Another man
cleared his throat several times in jest as he passed by us.
Thunder.

Try to forget. Say they're ignorant. If they knew, they'd feel bad. Whatever. I'm not sure what I'm expected to do. I live in this apartment, play games, watch videos. Attempt to motivate myself to keep smiling and laughing. But tonight I can't. It all seems bad. I've been here for almost four fucking months. Going to a movie is "an event." Grocery shopping and driving tire me out. Eating is a chore and none of my clothing fits. At this point I have no idea if I'll be at Brown in the fall. It seems unlikely.

The worst part is that what I'm waiting for will not fix me. Maybe I won't cough at the movies, but people will stare at me when I have a fat face. Maybe they'll even make fun of me. But I have no choices here. I just wish I could take a nap and wake up when lungs have been found. So much easier. 107 ccs have infused.

TURN OFF OLD PLANK ROAD

Drive for a while until an overgrown, unkempt driveway. Not marked, no warning. Easy to pass. Clearly it's been used before—see those skid marks? It's just wide enough for a modern-day family vehicle. Big stones cause bouncing, quick turns cause nausea. But at the bottom of the steep path lies relief.

There's the cabin with its wall of windows Dad and friends built, its roof we used to play on, the remnants of a lake view, a screened porch with tools and piles of old raincoats, a tall stack of mattresses in the main room, and an ever-expanding kitchen.

Smoke drifts from the chimney. Walk across the plank over the stream (it's often dried out in the summer) and begin to smell coffee and oatmeal, hear familiar voices, dread taking a trip to the outhouse.

I can't help thinking about that driveway. Seems scary when you first go down. Turn the wheel fast around this tree and that, try to avoid big rocks or muddy ruts in the way.

That's how I've lived all these years. Half knowing what to expect, yet realizing that over time it changes—it'll never be predictable. Won't even discuss how hard it is to go up. Talking about the driveway and going down it are different. With experience one feels the challenges instead of imagining them. But at least with the cabin's driveway I always know where it leads. I will never question what happens to me at the bottom, whom I will see again and whom I will not. I just want to put on the brakes, go back up, turn onto some other driveway, one that's paved, no surprises.

One that doesn't go down.

My Fears in My Seventeenth Year
(Now I'm Twenty)

Unsure when death will hit,
   (still am)
I don't want to sit in bed waiting for a transplant.
   (but I need to)
Will I be given the chance to pursue my childhood dreams?
   (Will I get to New Year's?)
Will I be halfway through college and have to give it up?
   (Will I get back to Brown?)

I don't want to sit in bed waiting for a transplant,
   (but I need to)
leashed to a tank of oxygen.
   (I don't wear O all the time)
Will I be halfway through college and have to give it up,
   (Will I get to Brown?)
forever frequenting the hospital?
   (whatever)

Leashed to a tank of oxygen,
   (I don't wear O all the time)
unable to travel to India or Australia,
   (So what? I can't even go home)

Forever frequenting the hospital—
   (whatever)

will I live at home when I should be away?
   (Will I ever get new lungs?)

Unable to travel to India or Australia,
   (So what? I can't even go home)
I don't want my busy friends to desert me.
   (It's not their fault. Besides, some haven't)
Will I live at home when I should be away,
   (Will I ever get new lungs?)
coughing up liters of blood?
   (It was half a liter last time)

I don't want my busy friends to desert me;
   (It's not their fault. Besides, some haven't)
I don't want to die alone,
   (I don't want to die before the transplant)
coughing up liters of blood.
   (It was half a liter last time)
What will happen to me when I die?
   (What will happen to me when I die?)

I don't want to die alone.
   (I don't want to die before the transplant)
Unsure when death will hit,
   (still am)
what will happen to me when I die?
   (What will happen to me when I die?)
Will I be given the chance to pursue my childhood dreams?
   (Will I get to New Year's?)

————————————————

Today is Lauren's day. God, I hope she wins the pool! Kat came up with this idea to create a betting pool around the date of my transplant, to make the wait less tedious. Bidders have been dropping like flies each day. Five people guessed July 4th, four guessed the 5th. I knew the holiday wouldn't yield lungs—too predictable.

Last Monday was another trip to Children's. We met Laurel at one P.M. by PFTs. She looked tan and refreshed after her two-week family vacation in the south of France. There was also a look of concern in her face when she saw me and I heard her tell Debra as they walked ahead later that we just need to find lungs. The PICC line had to come out, as I had suspected. I lasted for twelve days, ten of which were painful, but now the site was red, hot, and swollen.

The extraction is not a big deal, although Debra and Lauren seemed disturbed when they saw Laurel pulling out the 50-centimeter catheter. Because of the inflammation it was hard to get out. Tugging was involved at one point. And then a Band-Aid. Another closed-up hole.

What to do about my health? Oral antibiotics. Not a big deal. But wait. She wants me on Tobramyacin nebulizer treatments. I HATE them. Smelly, sticky—they take forever and they taste bad. To me it seems like an imposition. After all of it, do I really have to? I shrink, stop talking, expressing my discouragement by silencing myself.

Laurel went to pager headquarters to find me a new one that had legible numbers. Debra and Lauren went to Au Bon Pain for lunch and I sat in the garden. Sunny, breezy, quiet until a heli-copter lands overhead. Whenever I hear that noise I think of my lungs arriving at the hospital. If I see a cooler in the park I imag-ine my lungs inside of it. Driving to Providence a month ago I saw a truck labeled CASKET MAKERS. As if it were the same as bread or a mattress. Kept staring at the small square truck and swerving when I became too dazed.

Both my supporters vehemently opposed my desire to do away with Tobra nebs and were saddened. There is a unified belief by all those who love me that I should do every little thing to keep myself well no matter how much I hate it, no matter how miserable it makes me. But in this contained world even the smallest dislike becomes colossal since I'm accept-ing the bigger uncontrollable unpleasantries. I would not budge on this.

I saw Dr. Burr at 3:30. It was strange not being in Laura's little office anymore. I do miss her, or rather the comfort of having her there and knowing that she understood. Dr. Burr left for Mongolia yesterday and won't be back until the end of July. I've made an appointment for the 30th that I hope I won't be able to keep. If I become desperate I can see Laura in Newton, or call Dr. Raduns in New York, but it's not the same. On one hand I feel sort of cheated and abandoned. Everyone takes vacations, changes life goals, right when I need them. But on the other hand, I find it impossible to hold it against them. I am a patient of theirs, a part of the life, not a vital piece. I want them to live as they desire. I'm happy that Laura was able to move on. It's not easy to change daily activities after ten years.

I find myself torn about many things. It pleases me when friends call. However long it's been, however disconnected I feel, I know that it is an effort for them to pick up the phone, for them to hear about where my life is, and so it means something to me. After all, there are those who don't call or e-mail. And yet, a phone call ends by even those I feel closest to saying, "Well, I'll call next week." Or, "I'll be in Boston in the next couple weeks." And I realize that I am in a different time zone that very few are able to calculate.

In Between:
The Beginning

Phone rings. Half-dreaming, yet somehow knowing, I pick it up. "Hello?"

"Hi, Laura"—she pauses—"this is Laurel." Pauses again. "We have lungs." "You're kidding!" I say sleepily, realizing, as it comes out that of course she isn't.

"No, this is the real thing. It's still early, but so far everything is a go-ahead." And it all begins.

Jess, one of three friends from college visiting that weekend, wakes up in the bed across from me. She runs to what has become my parents' bedroom in this waiting room of an apartment. Kat and Emma start screaming and run in. I have an hour to get to the hospital. Planning for this day, staring at calendars, wishing, needing, in a city that wasn't mine, for four months. Hang up the phone.

Stay calm. Pick up the phone. Call my parents.

He picks up because the phone is on his side of the bed. "Hello?"

"Dad, we have lungs," I shout, half crying.

"You're kidding!"

"That's exactly what I said to Laurel." Chuckle.

I can hear him, "Mary, wake up, Mary, lungs."

Discuss details, but don't talk for too long—they have to get to Boston before the surgery begins. I'm sure I talked to Mom. I'm sure we said I love you.

Pick up the phone again. Call Debra, the godmother figure in my life. "I've got lungs."

"What? You got what? I'm on my way." She made it in one hour and fifty-seven minutes from Westchester. Luckily all the speeding cops were still asleep. Arliss, her husband, refuses to believe her time. In fact, most men won't believe it.

Pick up the phone again, continue to call down the list I'd made, just as I'm sure people do when a baby's on its way. I can't reach Lauren, who is away in D.C. for the weekend, but has been

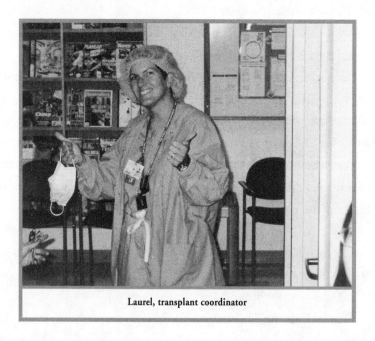

Laurel, transplant coordinator

living with me for the last month. Her cell phone isn't on. My former roommates are dressing, not sure how to help, very nervous. I finish the calls and get in the shower. If I'm about to go for this kind of thing I'd better wash my hair now and shave where I need to—who knows how long it'll be until I can take a real shower again. Professional patients have it down.

The hospital is silent. It's 6 A.M. on a Sunday. Laurel takes me to X ray—the last pictures of my lungs. I hold her coffee while she pushes the wheelchair. She's exhausted. Lots of work had to be done before I was even called. The whole time I keep hearing, "So far, everything looks good."

Minutes become hours. Get into the ICU bed, put on the gown, take all jewelry off, answer the same questions repeatedly, do some nebulizer treatments, and access my port-a-cath. Debra arrives; other friends come in pairs for short periods of time. Apparently the family waiting area is filling up with my visitors. They're tentatively taking me in at 11:30.

And then she's there. My mom. Exhausted and glowing all at once. Dad had sent her ahead in case I was on my way in. Despite an airline security strike on one of the shuttles they made it with about twenty minutes extra.

I am calm, excited, ready. But at a certain point my body begins to shake with fear. They give me Ativan. And the rest I remember with pictures. Finally, I was wheeled out of the ICU, all the friends who'd gathered surrounding me, giving me hugs, crying. We'd waited for this chance to stop death, begun to think it wouldn't arrive. My dad described how they took me into the elevator, everyone saying last wishes. I didn't look back.

Thus began our new life; my parents, the cat, and me. Gus

would spend most of the fall being fed by friendly doormen. I didn't know one surgery, after all these years of dealing with hospitals and illness, would change us all.

────────────────────

The day I woke everyone up.

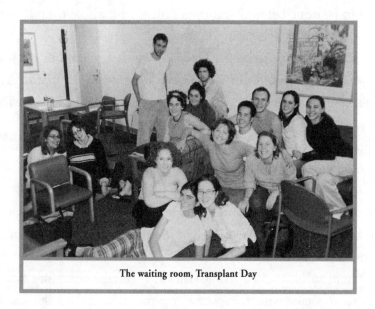

The waiting room, Transplant Day

Post-Transplant

No one can possibly know what is about to happen.
It is happening each time for the first time, for the only time.
—James Baldwin

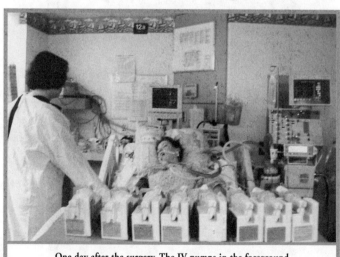

One day after the surgery. The IV pumps in the foreground
contain different medications.

I thought I was in London when I awoke five days later. Between the term bedspace for room and johnny for a gown all seemed, but then, well, it just didn't make sense. Why were all the doctors from Boston in a London hospital?

That Wednesday night I asked Debra, finally, after being confused all day: "Why did I have the transplant in London?"

"What?" And then she cleared things up.

JULY 29, 2001 ————————————————————

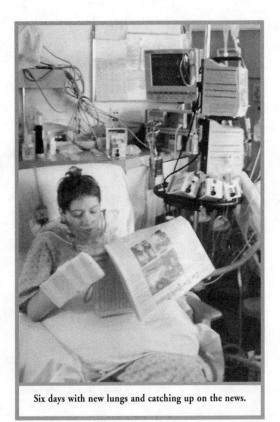

Six days with new lungs and catching up on the news.

Surgical fellow wakes me at 6:15. Two weeks ago I was already up, just arriving at the emergency room, waiting to be brought to the intensive care unit, cursing my cell phone because it wouldn't work that far into the ER. I had the paper to read, but didn't get much done.

I have a spot on my tank from last night's Japanese ginger dressing, and I'm covered in dry sweat from the change in temperature of this small eighth-floor room. And, let's be honest, it's 6:45 in the fucking morning, I should NOT be up at this hour! Couldn't care less. Get over others' norms, accept and relish in my own. It's quiet. Strung cranes sway in man-made air.

He listens to my lungs. I take deep breaths. Deep, deep, deep, like that Jersey Shore Ocean I miss dearly.

I can walk briskly down a hallway with my mother. And it'll only get faster. Aching left side will pass in a couple of days. It was re-sutured in the OR on Friday. It gushed blood for a couple days in a row. I would look down and then have a new red patch on my tank. Change the dressing. Still need that bit of a reminder—slow down, you just had a double lung transplant. Keep waiting and watching and imagining.

11:42 P.M. Okay, I WANT NON-DIET SODA!!!!!!!!!!!!

JULY 30, 2001 ————————————————————

5:30 Elwood wakes me. 8:00 Lillehei and Waltz. Just woken up, try to remember all the questions to ask before docs walk out. Maybe I could leave questionnaires for them to fill out instead. Go

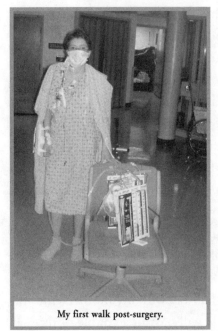

My first walk post-surgery.

through the plans. . . . GI consult for the diarrhea, more diabetes teaching, hopefully a new PICC line. Why is there so much phlegm? Keep up the chest PT, the coughalator, the walking.

In the ICU I was eager to shit in a toilet instead of on the bed. Now I've made it to the toilet, but I go in upside-down white plastic hats. The back one's for the diarrhea, the front for the pee. God forbid you forget to scoot back and forth and mistakenly mix them together. Then it can't be cultured. Yup, mine's so special it's going to be sent by U.S. postal to a special electron microscope in Toronto. I almost lost it when the Long Island GI fellow told me he had to look at my *heinie*. My what? I need to get a culture from your *heinie*. Okay, he's a dork. Sort of fun to be overly judgmental and make fun of all the people in and out.

And carbo-counting. It's going to be harder than I thought. My whole life I've just eaten. No worrying about fat or calories. I never look at labels or measure how many servings I'm eating. But it's better that than a restricted diet. I think I can handle a few shots a day.

Dad arrives for rounds every morning. He has tea from Au Bon Pain that never gets drunk. If I'm asleep he'll sit in the playroom across the hall reading the paper. We spend the mornings together, just like we took our walks to the Chapin bus stop. Laughing, bickering, loving.

AUGUST 1, 2001 ───────────────────

Mrs. Bonner and Lauren meet me in the garden—it's the place to be for lunch if you know anything about the hospital. Who would sit in the basement's cafeteria on a day like this? Round café-style tables line the side. All are filled at the peak hours, but we're a little later today (1:30) so it's starting to empty out. Settle at a table in the shade.

Eat my prosciutto sandwich from Zathmary's, the day before it was London broil. Yup, I'm in an extravagant mood. Drink my favorite Coke, all the while counting those carbs. Talk, talk, laugh, talk. BURP! It just came out. Head upon head simultaneously turns around to see who the culprit was, whispers, snickers. And the three of us couldn't stop laughing. I just had a lung transplant, sorry, I had to. Then we start making jokes about stool cultures and how mine went to Canada. The laughing gets worse.

One minute it is painful to cough, impos-

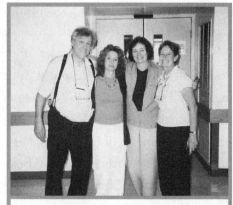

Part of Team Laura. My dad, my godmother Debra, my mom, and Mrs. O'Keefe.

sible to get anything up. Next I'm coughing and it rushes forth like the angry bull. This cough is different. It's a normal set of lungs trying to rid itself of stuff that shouldn't be there. They do not accept the phlegm. In fact, the right side feels so congested because the lungs are normal. What a feeling. I shouldn't be coughing at all. I don't cough. I don't feel like I have CF in my lungs. There isn't the same effort to breathe. Granted, there's wire holding my sternum together and that's a little heavy at times, but I don't need oxygen anymore.

Dinner time. Again, a Zathmary's buffet. More carbo-counting. The Bonners got me a book, though. It's a hand-held carbo-counter. Maybe cheating, but whatever, at least I now know how many grams of carbs are in falafel! Because I'll definitely be eating that a lot this fall. Father has decided we will take a Pepsi challenge. He numbers cups, pours in dark soda and Courtney and I take the test. We each sip, cup after cup, immediately saying how strange Three and Five are. Two is the favorite, Six is runner-up. And in the end, it's Pepsi One that wins, with Diet Coke right behind it. Pepsi and Coke were the first to go. I am mortified. I guess I can't complain about drinking diet soda anymore.

The rifabutin makes it harder for me to absorb the Neoral. My dose tonight is 750 mg. To put it in perspective, I started on 200 mg. Now I'm taking nine pills, seven of which are an inch long—they all smell like skunk. I was not happy about that last night. So I have my moments of frustration, but I think that's to be expected.

Today's EB's birthday. Happy Birthday, EB. EB's been one of my best friends since childhood. Her real name's Elizabeth, but in fifth grade I started calling her EB, which was occasionally her family's nickname.

AUGUST 2, 2001 ——————————————————————

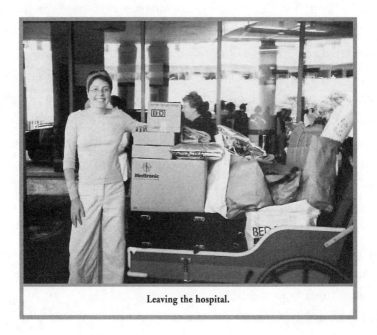

Leaving the hospital.

Sun's coming up. I can see her through the plastic shades just on the left side of the wall. I may go home tomorrow. Someone asked on the phone last night if I was nervous. NO. Excited more than anything to walk out of this building. Intrigued to see what will happen next. Hopeful that gradually I will gain more strength, that nebulizer treatments will be discontinued, that I will ride a bike.

AUGUST 5, 2001 ——————————————————————

Awake at 6 A.M. like I was three weeks ago, except now I'm home in bed, not rushing anywhere. Today I did not feel well.

Swollen. Gained five pounds in two days—puffed hands, sore ankles, and my face, well, just embarrassing. It looks like a medium-size pear. Hopefully Lillehei will put me back on Lasix tomorrow and I will feel less bloated.

Friday night I slept. Really slept, like I hadn't in awhile—no beeping pumps, no bloods drawn in the middle of the night. But in the morning I felt like I was right back in the ICU. I woke up in a pool of shit. Luckily it hadn't spread everywhere, but it had covered enough ground. Humiliating. Why hadn't I woken up? Feel like a combination of a baby who can't do things for herself and an old woman, too dignified to admit she can't do anything for herself. I want so badly to move with my new lungs, to bike and run and have energy, but I'm realizing that my body has yet to catch up. It will, but I have to be patient. After all this time waiting I just have to hold out a bit longer. I'm almost there. Now it's about rest and nurturing. Yet at times it's hard to remember that.

Tobra nebs, Pulmozyme, chest PT, pills. I'm still doing all those things, in fact, much more than I was before the transplant, but I don't mind. It's not futile anymore. Before a neb seemed like a waste of time. It wasn't going to make me well, or even feel better temporarily. Now there's a point to all of it. I know the pills work. I know the nebs are helping to get rid of the remaining secretions. I know that eventually I won't need as much medication and I will be active again.

The past few days have been hard. Wednesday was 8:30–3:30 at the hospital. Then Dad and I went down to Providence to look at my apartment, which was fun, but tiring.

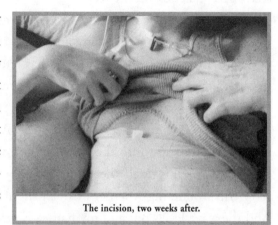

The incision, two weeks after.

Thursday I awoke incredibly sick to my stomach, NPO for the bronch (bronchoscopy). Wouldn't you know it, they overshot on the Neoral, my level was high, which left me shaky and nauseous all day long. Zofran did shit. We arrived in pre-op at noon. Moved to the isolation room in the recovery room at 1:30, then I was wheeled into the OR by about six people in blue I did not know at 2:45. Cynthia stopped by and we were able to chat and giggle for a bit before I went in. Dr. Dave stopped by, too.

But there was a sense of haphazardness that I would continue to experience later. Laurel was not there; Dr. Waltz was not there. I found myself reminding everyone what was supposed to happen. Don't forget to take out the chest tube stitches. Don't forget that my PICC line will need to come out afterward. How much Neoral should I take tonight? I was the only one who knew all the pieces. All the others were in charge of one area or another.

Shivering. Nausea. High blood pressure. It went on for hours.

I thought I would have to spend the night. And just when I was starting to get back on my feet.

Friday morning. Trembling hands so that it's hard to give myself insulin. At one point my arm starts to shake. Overnight I'd had diarrhea again. My old friend has returned. He took one day off, how kind. We buy Depends for overnight. Great. Now I'm wearing diapers.

Nausea. How do cancer patients do it? A two-hour car ride. I dry heave and spit into the New London water. A mid-storm ferry ride. Finally reach the house in Fisher's that I spent the ferry trip wondering whether or not I should have ventured to. And the wave levels out and my nausea is better. The cell phone conversation with Waltz earlier allowed me to skip the Neoral at night. But back on 700 mgs in the morning.

I sleep well in this princess room. Courtney and I always called it the strawberry room even though there are clearly small red tulips on the wallpaper and bigger ones to match on curtains and the rocking chair. I have a balcony. The air here is like the sea, taste the salt. Since 5:30 I've been turning. Pain sets in. Up at 7:30. Hug my new soft pillow for support, make faces, hope it'll pass. And then, in the bathroom, I see my face. It's finally arrived. Those cheeks I dreaded for so many months, the ones that make me look like a fat baby all over again, except not nearly as cute—I had strawberry blond hair and huge blue eyes. Now it's some thrown-together brown rug atop my head attached to a pear. And all this feeling so sick. I knew it wouldn't be as easy as it had been. There had to be a catch. It's not so bad. I'm not even discouraged. It's just that there are those moments when I look in the mirror, see myself, and my eyes tear. I hope that others can see past the external. More important, I hope that I can continue to see past it.

Subject: UPDATE

Date: Tue, 21 Aug 2001 22:25:33 -0400

From: Laura

SO, here is a VERY BELATED update:

Me and my new lungs are currently in the Brookline apartment. The past couple weeks have been a bit bumpy.

1) I was incredibly sick from one of the immunosuppressant medications called NEORAL, more commonly known as cyclosporine. Because of interactions with other medications I had to take 14 pills of that one medication a day, they're about an inch long each and they smell like skunk. NO, I AM NOT exaggerating! I was sick to my stomach and shaky most of the time. Yesterday they finally decided to switch me to another immunosuppressant called FK506. I'm already feeling better. That was the good news of the day!

2) My lung function, which had reached an amazing 95% at a certain point, has been steadily going down. It is now 78%. There seems to be something in my right lung and they aren't really sure what it is. Lots of guesses and technical words, but nothing concrete. I had lung biopsies done less than two weeks ago which did not show any rejection, so they don't think it's that. For this reason I have to have yet another bronchoscopy done on thursday august 24th. Then I'll have what's called a needle biopsy of my lung done on friday morning. I'll definitely be in the hospital thursday night, maybe over

the weekend, it's not clear just yet. Basically, it won't be a fun end to the week, but I'd like to start feeling a bit better.

3) In terms of my activity level, I was HOME this past weekend and got to see a good number of friends and family, although there are many I didn't get to see since I was only there for a few days. I'm up and about and trying my best to get my body back in shape, but that's going to take time especially since with low potassium I'm getting all these leg cramps—yuck.

4) I'm still hoping to be back at Brown come September 1st. Until that date I can be reached by e-mail or phone here in brookline hope all's well and please keep in touch. I've got these great new lungs and I want to use them as much as possible! (um, yeah, I like to talk a lot)

L

Subject: update e-mail
Date: Sat, 25 Aug 2001 08:50:39 −0400
From: Laura

SO, it's all over. I had my bronch and port placement thursday morning, then the needle biopsy yesterday morning and NO PNEUMOTHORAX (collapsed lung)! The biopsy results from the bronch show that I have acute bronchitis in my right lung. They only biopsy one lung, and the left one looks great so it's probably just the right one. Back on IV antibiotics. I have to stay here in the hospital at least until monday, but more results from other tests may come back so I may have to stay longer, we'll see. I hadn't been feeling well, though, so I was sort of expecting them to find something. And according to Dr. Waltz if they had to find something this was the way to go.

We'd much rather infection that's treatable than some kind of rejection!

In relation to my health I haven't gotten upset, but dealing with this hospital I'm sort of starting to lose it, at least I was thursday. There's SO MUCH bureaucracy here, so many people involved in my care, more when I'm doing things outpatient, and it gets frustrating . . . and stresses me out. Always feeling like I

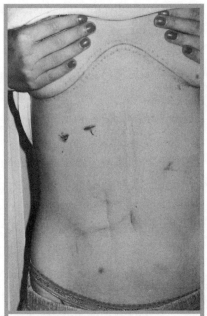

Four weeks after. The scar down the center is from an earlier surgery. The small incisions are from chest tubes, recently removed.

have to watch what others are doing to me because they probably won't think of this or that interaction. And I say that only because it's happened already.

I'm still trying to get back to brown at the end of the week. I can do home iv, so it's not an unrealistic plan. Trying to go with the flow. Cell phone's the best way to reach me or e-mail . . .

AUGUST 26, 2001 ─────────────────────────

Before, coughing was like breathing should be—my body did it without any effort. Now it's uncomfortable. Just brought up a slug plug. Really, the consistency, color, everything reminds me of slugs we'd find when I was ten stuck to Molly's walkway in Palisades. Vital signs were at 6:30. I can't get back to sleep.

Six weeks. Doesn't sound like a long time, but it feels like years. Kenny is on bypap in the ICU. He was transferred down there yesterday. It's eerily quiet on the floor now that he isn't coughing away. If it doesn't work he'll be intubated and then, well, I already think it's over. He had a liver transplant in February and now he's dying six months later. He's only fifteen. I can't help but feel guilty. One of the hardest parts about this transplant is that I feel like I should be grateful for every second, you know? Like if I'm not then I don't deserve these lungs. But I guess I just have to realize that I'm allowed to get upset about dealing with post-transplant issues, too.

I'm sick of peeing in upside-down hats. I'm sick of being in the hospital, always watching what goes in and how much. I've already caught several mistakes: glucose in the IV meds, Vanco levels being drawn through my central line. I haven't been stressed about my health lately, just dealing with hospital bureaucracy.

I wonder what will happen if this cavity is cepacia, whether that will matter. I guess I'll find out in the next couple days. Whatever the verdict I'll be doing home IV for sure at least for the first couple weeks of school, if not the whole month of September. Could be worse, I could be stuck in the hospital.

AUGUST 28, 2001, 12:20 A.M. ─────────

Dark, quiet, stare at the ceiling, touch my slowly keloiding scar. Not allowed to have my fan on because it hasn't been approved by biomed. Yeah, it's going to burn down the hospital because it only has two prongs. Another rule determines. It's tiresome. My left eye keeps twitching and my pupils are dilated but that doesn't seem to bother anyone else.

All this talk about can or can't I head back to Brown. And I wonder what else I'm supposed to do. I'm tired of asking permission—can I go to the garden? Can I get Benadryl IV and sleep through the night? No, of course not. Why let her sleep? Certainly it matters more that it be given by mouth than that she get eight hours of rest. And, well, we can't find another antibiotic to put her on. Who gives a shit if Zosyn will cause diarrhea. And the shakiness, well she has to be on either Neoral or Prograf and we know she prefers the Prograf.

Subject: big bump
Date: Sun, 02 Sep 2001 14:59:33 −0400
From: Laura

This will be a pretty impersonal e-mail—for that I am sorry.

On Tuesday I went to Brown to register—I got to leave the hospital for the day. But that night I started having abdominal pain. It got worse and worse and the nausea began. By the next morning I was vomiting for five hours. They did an x ray and a ct scan and put a tube down my nose. I was taken into surgery Wednesday night to correct my small bowel obstruction—it lasted for several hours.

Since the surgery I have been in a lot of pain and nauseous practically all the time. I haven't really been talking on the phone because I feel too sick. I'm on TPN and Intralipids to keep

my nutrition up and I'm on so many things by IV that I have a
port and a picc line. I'm walking in the halls a bit now, but it's
still hard. Until I "pass gas" I'm not allowed to eat or drink.
Basically it's just bad luck. Abdominal surgery, which I had in
tenth grade, is hellish. Just bad luck. The hope is that once my
bowels start moving the recovering will speed up. I feel like it's
been years, but it's only been four days. Keep in touch. The
truth is that this has been way harder than the transplant, a big
bump if you will. But I'm still trying, trying, trying to get well.

　all my love,

　Laura

SEPTEMBER 8, 2001 ————————————

Sometimes you just want it to stop. You just want to ask God
or whoever is up there to give you a break. And I don't think I've
done that. I don't think that I've really truly complained this
whole time, this whole ordeal. I may have said I was in pain or
last week pleaded to stop the nausea, crying . . . but I went
through it. And I'll continue because I have no choice.

But today, for the first time in a while, I felt more like myself,
as if I'd emerged from an underwater trek, a post-op narcotic-
induced haze. The FK level, the amount of a certain immunosuppressant (FK506) in my body, was back down from toxic
levels, my renal function was, not good, but better than the day
before. Then the cramping came this afternoon—I have a diff. A
bacterial bowel infection. Okay, I can deal. I can go on. Just a

couple more pills. After all, with the kidneys not functioning well they'd already stopped most other drugs.

But, to flush out the kidneys I need two liters of fluid in me, not allowed any Lasix. My face has puffed up, my eyelids are swollen, my fingers swollen once again and my chest has fluid in it as well. It hurts in my sternum when I cough. In fact, it's not even a cough, more like a cat wheeze. How pathetic.

Fell asleep at 11:30. Bob had to give me my Ampho neb when I was fast asleep. Suddenly gasping, pain, feels like I can't breathe. And I lose it. Enough, I say, enough. So what's the price I have to pay for being given these lungs? Is it that if I suffer enough at a certain point I will have proven I want to live? Is it like that? Oh because if it is, whoever's spirit left this world, I do want to live, I do, I do. Thank you, thank you. I will never be able to repay you. And I guess for that reason I can't complain. I don't deserve to. I am lucky to have these lungs. Yet it's September 8, one in the morning and I'm still in this fucking Red Sox territory. I know there's no deadline for recovery, but for each and every part of my body to be at peace, to work together—will it ever happen?

Subject: checking in
Date: Tue, 11 Sep 2001 20:46:30 −0400
From: Laura

AGAIN, a massive e-mail.

What a day I imagine all have had. I watched it unfold while getting chest pt, just in disbelief as the twin towers crashed down one by one. I hope that all friends and family of friends are safe.

I just wanted to let you know that I will be in the hospital for a few more days. I packed everything up today to head home, we even made it to the car when a resident came out to tell us there was a controversy over my latest biopsy results. Wouldn't you know it I have what's called stage 2 rejection. Luckily it's treatable. Unfortunately it's only treatable with VERY HIGH DOSES of IV steroids, so I don't think I'll feel all that well in the next couple days, may be a bit moody, we'll see.

Again, hope all hanging in and sorry to add a little more not so great news to the day, but this is just another bump.

all my love,

Laura

Subject: guess where I am?!
Date: Tue, 18 Sep 2001 08:59:47 −0400
From: Laura

SO . . .

I am FINALLY back at Brown. Well, I have been since Sunday. I got out of the hospital on friday after 22 days, actually longer than I was there for my transplant! The last few days of high-dose steroids were not as bad as expected, although my face is quite, shall we say, full. I will be in boston tonight until friday because I have another bronch on thursday. But then I will be returning to providence. It's good to be back here. Of course, there will be adjustment, but it feels right.

I apologize for not responding to e-mails, but each and every one has helped me tremendously. I wasn't talking a lot

in the hospital after the surgery, and during the steroids I
needed more than ever to keep things in to prevent myself
from losing it.

I hope this e-mail finds you relatively well despite all that
seems to be changing around us.

all my love,

Laura

Subject: it's neverending
Date: Thu, 04 Oct 2001 07:47:10 −0400
From: Laura

Bad news.

My pulmonary function is not improving. The doctors
believe that I have more rejection. I am having ANOTHER
bronch in a couple hours, then I will be in the hospital in
boston AGAIN for a few days to get the VERY high dose
steroids. This is "round 2" of the steroids. If I do not improve
after this there will be a "round 3" and then, well, they try
something stronger. I've been back and forth between providence and boston the past couple weeks. I am happy to be
back at brown, yet having a hard time. I'm just not as well as I
want to be and I don't know whether I will get better or . . .
I'm not trying to be melodramatic, this has been what I am
thinking about the most in the last couple days. Hopefully the
next e-mail will be a bit more cheerful. Keep in touch.

off to shower!

Laura

COLUMBUS DAY WEEKEND ——————

East 66th. Mom bakes Nana's seasonal Concord grape pie. The leftover pulp sits in a glass pitcher in the fridge. It has a jelly center, a butter crust. Outdated pictures and books never read, piles of unsorted stuff from Boston, and there's Ellie whom I'm not allowed to sleep with anymore on my stuffed animal pile. Reassuring excess, warm pink, drawers with clothes I "was wondering where that was." Return with an extra bag from New York. A man rides by me on a unicycle. Another has a great floppy dane.

Subject: hi from home
Date: Sun, 07 Oct 2001 09:50:36 −0400
From: Laura
  To: a friend
  hey
  so high-dose steroids ended yesterday morning and I flew
with dad on the USair shuttle to nyc. It is SOOOOOOOOOO good
to be home! I can't even tell you. . . . I saw a friend yesterday
and did window shopping and of course had to stop into
bloomies which was a madhouse! I'm going to Shun Lee Cafe for
dim sum today—yum, yum, yum! I think I'll be here until thursday when I'll fly back to boston for the bronch on friday. I must
get my eyebrows done on thursday. . . . it's getting embarrassing! I'm feeling a bit better but still skeptical as to whether this
second round of steroids did much. How are things up there?

Is it cold in boston because it is fucking FREEZING here. Luckily I

left some sweaters in nyc so I can stay warm.

LOVE YOU

L

——————————————

It's so easy for people to hang up the phone. And I can't. They hear the story, they sympathize, offer to help, and then I don't talk to them for a week. All these names and faces and then it's just me. Again and again I come back to that and I'm not sure why it bothers me.

It's been three months. And I hear myself say that and it's supposed to be a long time. But in the grand scheme of a life, it isn't. Yet in three months so much has happened to my body I'm not sure I even know it. There was one body before the transplant and one after. And I don't think you can go through something like that without it affecting your mind. Who am I now?

Yet this milestone is not what it was expected to be. I'm still at the hospital every week, getting bronchs, about to be readmitted for rejection therapy. I walk up the stairs and can't breathe. When I cried today I started coughing just like before—hacking, even though I don't have the same nerves to feel my lungs.

And no one remembered. Not even Mom. It's not their fault, people lead busy lives. I need to be strong enough to be happy on my own and I'm just not. I'm not. I very much believe right now that I don't have a future, that I'll be lucky if I get five years. Maybe I'm overreacting. And being lonely now, not feeling like I have many friends around to lean on just leaves me here on this Monday night, crying to myself and wondering what I should do. I have to do my IV dose. My ampho neb. My vital signs. All in my night's routine. Deep down I just want someone to call out of the blue, just to check on me. I better not wait up for it.

Subject: update
Date: Fri, 19 Oct 2001 11:22:03 –0400
From: Laura

SO, here is the news.

On Wednesday my doctors said that they believe I have chronic rejection. Not what we were hoping for. They are still saying that because it is so early on maybe my pfts will go back up again. I came into the hospital yesterday (in boston) to start what's called ATG (anti-thymocyte globulin). The medication is given everyday and runs in for 4–6 hours. The idea is that it will kill all my T-cells and then when more t cells grow back they won't have figured out that the lungs aren't mine. My first dose yesterday was not fun. I got chills, aching in my legs, a horrific headache and then pain all up and down my back—and this was despite being pre-treated with tylenol and benadryl. They ended up not completing the first dose because they said that I didn't need to be this mis-erable and they would find stronger pre-treatments for me. It was hellish. I can't even begin to think about doing this for two weeks if it doesn't get better, but they have reassured me it will. And if it works, if it sets the rejection back, it'll be worth it.

   NOW, there is a not so positive side to all of this. If we can't get the pfts back up, we're right back where we were before. Chronic rejection won't go away and it'll mean treatments and hospitalizations to push it back if we can. It could be slow or fast. I'm hopeful this stuff will work, but I'm also realizing it might not. I love you all so much and hope that things are going well for you. You can reach me by e-mail or cell.

   Laura

OCTOBER 22, 2001 ——————————————————

Here I sit knitting my fourth hat. I'm also working on Will's damn scarf which seems as if it will never be finished. I think it's been in progress for over a year now. It's 5:30 in the hospital, days are getting shorter and so the hospital becomes quieter earlier. My cozy lamp light is on and my fingers work meticulously with these small needles. This hat is made out of thin wool so it will take longer.

The ATG is going in. Neck is sore, head aches, hot. And shaky today, not sure why, but more tremulous.

Thursday night's dose was pure hell. I could feel the medication in me, my body fighting the antibodies, the antibodies killing the T-cells. Every part of me was at war. And people talk so much of metaphorical war with illness, but it did feel like I was being attacked. And I kept telling myself that it's to make me feel better. To get better. But I kept saying that I couldn't do it for two weeks.

"Mommy, I can't do this for two weeks."

And she knew it and I knew it and thank god for the sol-umedrol that has made the reactions minute in comparison. Now I'm blah and in the evenings my eyes droop like a basset hound as I try to stay awake until 11 P.M. I'm not sure why but there's something about that time that I feel like it's acceptable for me to go to sleep as a twenty-year-old. I mean, it's early for most, but it feels just late enough. The uncertainty fills room 822 and I wait to find out my fate, just as I waited for lungs just over three months ago. It's quiet. So quiet.

OCTOBER 25, 2001

Today is my parents' twenty-sixth wedding anniversary. Does a bronch represent a bad year to come? Or maybe a bad year past? It was not fun today. Dr. Jones irrigated my sinuses and I was in immense pain when I awoke. I agreed to morphine, which resulted much later in itching and nausea. I was in and out of sleep all afternoon, my father has a cold and couldn't be with me and, well, now it's 11 P.M. and I'm still scratching. My throat was sore for hours. I just kept asking for Mott's applesauce.

Shawna and Kelly sat outside on chairs for a while. Shawna's on oxygen and Kelly gets wheezy, but they're both so cute. I mean, four years younger, but something sweet about them both. I can tell even though I'm the baby in transplant that they look up to me. And it helps me as well to speak with them. Swap stories and complain about doctors.

Dr. Waltz is encouraged by my progress. I'm glad *he* is. Am I

too negative? I just don't want to get my hopes up. PFTs have
gone up a bit and everyone rejoices. But I want longevity, not one
little hill. Once it lasts I'll be pleased. And it's great that I won't
be having a bronch next week, that now I can go at least two
weeks, but still, even that, if I really think about it, please.
Relatively things are getting a bit better. Slowly we're crossing
problems off the list, but anesthesia every other week is still not
okay. A new nodule in my left lung leaves me uneasy, even if
Waltz isn't concerned. And I'm still getting out of breath when I
walk around—what's up with that? I have a good few days, but if
I think about all of it, the future, it becomes bleak. So we focus
on the small victories, I guess.

Subject: DETAILED UPDATE
Date: Sun, 28 Oct 2001, 17:43:12 –0500
From: Laura

So, once again I send an update. I have been silent for a
couple days but not without reason. Thursday I had my
bronch. The GOOD NEWS is that things "looked better" in
there, meaning that there was not as much scar tissue
buildup, not as much infection in the right lung, so the verdict
was that I was finally able to be taken off my IV Vancomycin
(after at least six weeks or so) and that we can probably start
going to at least every other week bronchs if not less fre-
quently. In perspective this is very exciting.

As a favor to me, my ENT guy here, Dr. Jones, irrigated my
sinuses while I was under anesthesia (saves me a trip to his
office which just hasn't gotten done since the transplant).

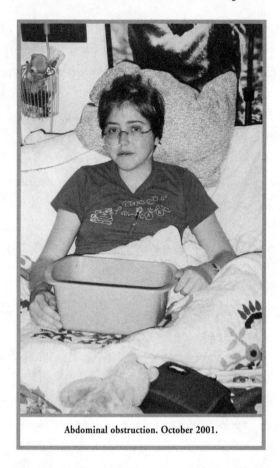

Abdominal obstruction. October 2001.

However, as a result I was in a LOT of pain on thursday after-noon. For some reason I agreed to take morphine for the pain, which left me nauseous and itchy all day long—not much fun. By thursday night, though, I was more myself, but, my tummy started to hurt . . . . . .

And, well, haven't we seen this scenario before?

By Friday afternoon I was in much more abdominal discom-fort and they started me on something called golytely, the joke being that it's not supposed to make you "go lightly" at all. Well, it didn't work, and only caused more pressure to build up in my abdomen. By Friday evening I had already had three unsuccessful enemas and the nausea was under way. The vomiting bile started later at night and I was pretty much up most of the night. Surgery was called in, there were lots of KUB x-rays (stands for kidney, urinary tract I think, bowel—could be wrong about those initials), a three am abdominal ultrasound with a very nice radiology fellow who was wearing a brown t-shirt and me yelling at what I named "the surgery guy" who didn't seem to be making a whit of difference with pain in the middle of the night. The tests showed that my large intestine was "full" and my small intestine had some blockages as well, although not as bad as last time.

Friday morning I had something called a gastrografin enema, which I barely remember except that it managed to clear out the large intestine. And finally, thanks to mucomist through my nose tube (that was put in Friday evening) there was, well, "the bowel movement heard round the hospital" at about four am today (sunday). The nose tube came out this morning. I'm still drinking mucomist every so many hours and it gives me bad abdominal cramping, but I am a new woman compared to yesterday. I was very close to having surgery again. Someone or thing was watching over me and pulled me through. Truth is I have no clue how I made it through the last couple days because it was just such hell again. But you wouldn't know it if you saw me today!

And, as for the rejection, well, that has taken a back burner with all else going on. Up until today I was getting the

ATG and tolerating it well. My t-cells are gone and my white count is holding. They'd like me to stay on it if I can for a full fourteen days.

Unfortunately they've found some kind of nodules on my ct scan, three to be exact, the largest being at the base of the left lung about the size of a marble. They don't know what they are. I'm having another ct guided needle biopsy on tuesday at 2 pm. However, I don't have to stay in the hospital to await results from that. I think, and this is a big THINK, that I will be leaving the hospital on wednesday or thursday, but of course, anything can happen between now and then.

I apologize for all the room confusion. I did end up moving rooms and am in 818, or my cell, of course.

all my love,

Laura

Subject: what to say . . . .
Date: Tue, 30 Oct 2001 23:05:58 −0500
From: Laura

GOOD NEWS

my abdominal obstruction is BETTER. They still have me on a liquid diet and I'm still taking the dreadful mucomist four times a day. I was FINALLY feeling more like myself today when I went for the needle biopsy. . . . .

The nodule in my lung is at the base of the left lung and it was very hard for them to biopsy it because every time I breathe it moves. Sort of like trying to hit a constantly moving target. SO, I was down in ct scan, half sedated with a needle in the lung and all of a sudden there is a lot of pain and wouldn't you know it I got a pneumothorax, which means, for those who don't know, that my lung collapsed. Then they put in a chest tube for drainage. It would have just been a minor complication had they actually gotten tissue to biopsy, now the whole thing becomes frustrating.

It's not definite, but at some point tomorrow I will probably be going to the operating room so that they can biopsy this nodule. They will try to go in with a scope as opposed to doing a complete open lung biopsy but they are unsure whether that will be possible until they get in there. Regardless, there will probably be a lot of pain for several days and it'll take several weeks of recuperation. I will be in the hospital through the weekend at least. I had the option of waiting several weeks to do the biopsy but I decided I'd rather get it over with now. I'm already here, I'm already in pain, I want to know what is causing this thing to grow . . . . my health comes first and so waiting doesn't make sense. That's the deal. I'm not going to write more because I'm pretty drugged (had codeine and percocet) and I'm not quite sure how coherent this e-mail is.

Yesterday I had a bit of a breakdown and so I've been pretty good today. Of course it seems like things just keep going wrong, but I don't seem to be given more than I can handle at least not so far . . . . . . keep in touch

all my love,

Laura

Subject: latest news from hospital central
Date: Mon, 05 Nov 2001 22:18:00 −0500
From: Laura

It's been about a week since the last update and a lot has happened. On Halloween they took out the nodule in my left lung and did a tiny wedge resection of the lung which basically means that they biopsied the lung. Doing it surgically they were able to get a bigger sample than they usually get in the bronchs. The surgery took four and a half hours and I was in a lot of pain afterward until they put me on a high enough amount of pain medication through the epidural (small catheter for pain inserted into the spine for those who don't know). That just came out yesterday and I am now on oral painkillers. The switch is always hard and I need a lot of pain stuff by mouth in the beginning, so I was a ZOMBIE today— just drugged out, kind of funny.

I'll go with the good news first . . . . . .

So far there is not vascular chronic rejection as they had feared there would be in the biopsy from the lung. This means that the rejection I have been experiencing is more of the short-term kind or maybe that the ATG which I just spent two weeks getting has helped. It does not mean we are free from dealing with rejection or anything of the sort but it is much better to have this result than to have my lungs filled with chronic rejection.

But, after the last couple months it is almost comical that I write the next paragraph. The pathology results from the nodule are not so good. I have been diagnosed with what is called POST TRANSPLANT LYMPHOPROLIFERATIVE DISEASE.

THE WAY I GOT IT: My body was unable to fight a virus (probably the epstein-barr virus which is the one that causes mononucleosis, although they aren't sure at this point) because of all the immunosuppression I am on. As a result, the virus has caused clumps of b-cells to grow into nodules and these in turn are making me sicker, possibly adding to the decline in the pfts.

WHAT IT IS: Another damn complication! It is NOT cancer, although oncology is the service that knows the most about it because it has to do with the lymph nodes and they will be helping to make decisions about which kind of treatment is best for me. I don't know yet exactly what they will decide for treatment, but I will hopefully find that out in the next couple days.

TREATMENT: The best thing they could do for me would be to stop all immunosuppressants, but they can't do that because that will cause outright rejection.

1) They have, however, lowered my immunosuppression medication doses. And there will be a fine line between too low and not low enough—it's very complicated.

2) There is a medication that will sort of turn off the switch to the cells that are growing like crazy. It's an IV med—rituximab. They will probably start me on that although I am not sure yet. And I don't know how often it is given or what the side effects are yet.

3) There is a chance I may be put on some kind of chemotherapy, but that is slim. They did do ct scans today to see if there are nodes anywhere other than my lungs—I don't know the results of those yet.

SO, basically I have this diagnosis and I'm waiting for all the right minds to come together and make a decision plan—that will hopefully be in the next couple days. And hopefully they will start whatever treatment it is this week. I'm scheduled for a bronch on friday and should be here in the hospital through then, although I'm planning to speak at Louella's interfaith dinner at brown on thursday night (I can get a Leave Of Absence from the hospital for a few hours). I will be spending thanksgiving at home in new york and hope to make it back to providence before then.

I don't know yet what this means long term for the lungs—I don't have that sense at the moment. I'm still very much in business mode, trying to figure this new thing out and understand what I have to do to feel better.

off to bed

all my love,

Laura

NOVEMBER 6, 2001

Well, it's just about midnight and today was Election Day. I sent in my absentee ballot a couple weeks ago. Truth is I have no clue who'll be a better mayor. I'm barely in New York at the moment anyway.

I made myself a snack at the patient nourishment center down the hall. The transplant floor is stocked with certain kinds of food. Never any salt because it's bad for renal patients—we all have to suffer. There's Swiss Miss pudding and Jell-O and popsicles in the fridge, not to mention an abundance of apple juice and cranberry and both milk percentages. Then we've got Campbell's chicken noodle soup, peanut butter, sliced bread, graham crackers, and my personal favorite—the Unsalted Premium Saltines. Those things are addicting. Lastly there are the individual cereal packs. Right now we're stocked with Cheerios, Raisin Bran, and Rice Krispies. I only eat the latter in treat form. But I mix the first two every morning for breakfast.

I've cut down on drinking so much apple juice since I found out that it's not supposed to be good for motility. I'm REALLY working hard at this bowel thing now. Apple juice was one of my staple post-transplant drinks. Oh, there's also free soda on the floor—Coke, ginger ale. That's a huge plus. I do, however, miss the cheddar cheese packs they used to have at Columbia. Here they have cheap slices of American. The kitchen on the floor has a toaster. We fought endlessly senior year to try to get one in the cafeteria at Chapin, but the administration was too afraid we'd burn the place down. Here they're more concerned about hanging lights in my room than trouble with a toaster.

Tonight I made myself some toast and loaded on the butter. Back to drinking Snapple lemon iced tea and my sugars aren't happy with me. I stuck myself at least six or seven times today to try to keep my sugar within range and I wasn't even that successful. Diabetes is the cherry on the transplant sundae. If I'm having a bad day it's frustrating. I don't want to be my pancreas for the rest of my life. Okay, fine, if I'm playing soccer and going to classes I can deal with sticking myself and taking pills, all of it. But these past few months have not even come close and it doesn't seem as if I'm going to get much of a relief before the new year, either. Starting to fall asleep. I'll write more tomorrow.

Subject: talked to the docs . . . . .
Date: Wed, 07 Nov 2001 14:34:05 −0500
From: Laura
To: a friend

LATEST NEWS hot off the presses just for you!

I left some babbling message on your house machine last night . . . . . god, I feel so stupid when I leave messages knowing that there is the possibility that so many people will hear them . . . . . whatever . . . . . do they know about me and the hospital? I hope so or everything must sound even weirder.

SO, they are going to hold off on doing a bone marrow biopsy which I am happy about. I've heard they're pretty painful and that your hip is sore for a while. This afternoon I will be getting a blood transfusion because my red cells have been low (very anemic) and I've been very short of breath and they're hoping this will help. I don't think it's such a big deal but I haven't had one when I was alert before, just in 1981 when I was a baby and during the transplant.

Then, after the transfusion, I will be getting the rituximab, which is "the treatment" for the lymphocyte disorder. My guess is that the first dose will make me sick, just like the ATG did—chills, aching, nausea, headache, fevers. But we'll see . . . . . there is always the chance I won't react. I think it's an eight-hour infusion. After today's I have three more to go, one a week. We'll do a ct scan then and hopefully the nodules will be gone. If they are, GREAT, although there is the chance they'll come back. If they're not gone then we move on to some kind of chemotherapy. Let's hope we don't have to go there, too, or at least not before christmas. I'm sorry that you won't be in new york for thanksgiving, but I totally understand why. I just hope I get to see you for more than a few minutes in december.

Some friends from brown are coming up for dinner tonight, so that should be fun, even though I probably won't be feeling too well. And then tomorrow night I'm taking that leave of absence to go down to brown and speak at louella's interfaith dinner. I hope I don't start crying when I'm talking . . . .

love you and talk to you soon,

Laura

Subject: [Fwd: Thursday Supper]

Date: Thu, 08 Nov 2001 09:53:29 −0500

From: Louella Hill

Greetings All!

We hope the week has gone well for each of you, and if it hasn't, the weekend is nearly here. We would like to invite you to this week's (Interfaith) Thursday Supper. Tomorrow, we will be joined by a very special guest. Fellow student Laura Rothenberg will talk about what it means to live with a serious illness. (Because of Laura's health, it would be best for any-one who is sick with a cold or the flu to not attend this week.) She was diagnosed with Cystic Fibrosis at 3 days old, and now today struggles to stay a student at Brown. Her story will undoubtedly be touching.

Thursday Supper is held every week at 58 Keene Street. All are welcome and invited to attend. Dinner is served at 5. Vegetarian options are always available. Kosher meals are available upon request. The talk will conclude by 7. To get there, walk through Faunce Arch toward Pembroke. Walk for 8 blocks, turn right, the house is the third on your left. The dog is named Fenway.

Thursday Supper is sponsored by the Office of the Chaplains and Religious Life at Brown University. For more information, please contact one of us (but please, do not hit reply—this is a listserv).

Until then, be in peace—

Love,

Heidi and Lou

Subject: leaving the hospital
Date: Sat, 10 Nov 2001 14:55:36 −0500
From: Laura

so, this will be a quick e-mail . . . . .

Yesterday was the first dose of the rituximab (treatment for the lymphoproliferative disease). I will get three more doses, each a week apart in the next few weeks. Unfortunately, in part from the LPD and then for reasons unknown, maybe some rejection, they aren't sure, my pft's have gone down tremendously (now only 38%) so I'm not feeling very well—a fair amount of shortness of breath. However, I have decided to leave the hospital and head back to providence until wednesday when I'll come back to brookline and have a bronch on thursday, then the next rituximab dose on friday. Then I will be in new york for thanksgiving week.

It's very frustrating to be leaving the hospital with oxygen and not feeling well, but I am hopeful that eventually this new medication will start to work against the nodules in the lungs and then my lung function will go back up. It's going to take time, though. It hasn't been the cheeriest few days, but I think being out of the hospital will help and if I start to feel worse I can always come back.

keep in touch,

Laura

Subject: latest news from Laura
Date: Wed, 14 Nov 2001 09:24:30 −0500
From: Laura

where to start . . . . .

I DID leave the hospital on Saturday. Mom and I went to the supermarket to stock up on all those things Abby doesn't eat (hot dogs, turkey, root beer). Down to Providence. We arrived, she unpacked and took the train back to New York.

Abby had a very nice dinner at the apartment for me, (my

good friend) Louella cooked a delicious squash meal and despite the fact that I was not feeling well and on oxygen, it was great—lots of people around all evening.

Of course I did spend half my evening going back and forth between Hasbro children's hospital and the CVS in east providence to fill my pain medication prescription that they'd failed to give me in Boston. Because it's a narcotic the resident had to find someone in RI who would write the prescription and give it to me and then I had to deliver and pick it up myself. Anyway, that was a pain. . . .

Sunday I had a nice brunch with Kat, Jess and Emily and then did some errands. But it was becoming increasingly harder for me to breathe and I was becoming more and more uncomfortable. At this point I had pretty much made the decision in my head that I was going to come back into the hospital on monday. Sunday evening I had dinner in with Abby Greenbaum and watched movies (Legally Blonde and The Big Lebowski) and arranged with Dr. Waltz to come into the hospital monday and have the bronch tuesday instead of waiting until the end of the week.

Well, wouldn't you know it, my belly, which had been hurting all day long, was not getting better. It was bloated and I was getting cramping pains just like with the other obstructions. I tried to go to bed, but finally around 3 am I woke abby up (I was nauseous at this point) and said we had to go to the ER. SO, my saving grace roommate popped out of bed, took all my stuff down to the car and drove me to boston at 3:30 in the morning. And she stayed with me for twelve hours until my dad got there. I could not have done it without her. When we were driving up, the moon was exquisite. A large, dangling hammock, or a big smile, whatever you want to call it.

The time in the ER was long and exhausting and somewhat unproductive. They did an abdominal CT eventually and just found that I was super backed up AGAIN. They've stopped my pain medication now and keep hammering me with the mucomist and we're just going to have to "watch my sluggish intestines VERY carefully." The downside of that is that my left lung is still in a lot of pain from the nodule removal two weeks ago, so tylenol will have to do, I guess.

And yesterday I had the bronch I had arranged for. AND, wouldn't you know it, I was RIGHT, and there was narrowing in both lungs, more so in the right middle bronchus. That one they had to dilate a couple of times and behind it they found lots of secretions, so I'll probably be on iv antibiotics. I'm not feeling AS short of breath, although I'd be lying if I said it was all gone.

And today, well, I'm just here in the hospital, in a fairly ok mood. I'm getting my next rituximab dose probably thursday and who knows when I'll head back to new york. I'm glad that I tried to go back to providence. I think maybe it just wasn't the right time, a little too sick, but it was worth it. I'm only sorry that I didn't get to see more friends.

all my love,

Laura

room 820

Subject: take me back to manhattan

Date: Tue, 20 Nov 2001 01:11:37 -0500

From: Laura

It's definitely bedtime, but before that I just wanted to send a pre-holiday health update.

LUNGS: It was a very good idea that I insisted the bronch be done on tuesday instead of thursday because they found that airways in both lungs were scarred, which meant increased narrowing and that was causing me to have so much trouble breathing. The biopsies revealed no acute rejection so that's GOOD news and after a couple days of deliberations they've decided not to keep me on iv antibiotics—also nice. Although the dilation (where they put the little balloons in the airways to open them up) did help, my pfts have only increased to 42%. Doesn't look like we're going to be back in the sixties quite yet, but the important part is that I'm feeling better and not aware of my breathing all the time like I was. I just get out of breath when I'm moving around.

TUMMY: Although I did not have a blockage when I came to the ER early monday morning (a week ago) I was incredibly backed up. All this past weekend I got what's called "golytely" through an NG tube, after several failed enemas earlier in the week. They had to give me six liters of the stuff. That's a lot—I think a usual adult dose is about two liters. And I still wasn't completely cleared out. But finally today dr. lillehei took pity on me and said enough is enough and, well, hopefully we've made room for turkey and all the other good food I'm planning to have this week in new york.

PTLD: Got my rituximab on thursday and once again I toler-
ated it well. The next dose will be given on wednesday in new
york at my good old hospital—columbia in the outpatient clinic
and genevieve and rechelle have promised not to neglect me
too much ☺ Still having night sweats and that's just a symp-
tom of the disease, so oh well.

oh yes, of course there's always something NEW: I spent
my weekend dealing with these strange and uncontrollable
shaking episodes. Courtney's mom, Ann O'Keefe, was here
with me and was a great help. And Lauren came by to pitch
in as well. Vicki visited earlier in the week. And Debra was
here for the last day. Some of them were horribly violent
shakings but they've calmed down now that they have me
on ativan several times a day at a low dose. However neurology was consulted and I had a head ct, an mri of my head
and two eeg tests where they put all the electrodes on your
head with this gross stuff and then it's almost impossible to
get it out of your hair. I looked like frankenstein especially if
you add the nose tube to it and then the heart monitor during the episodes and the oxygen for the worse ones when I
would get really out of breath. But now, as I said, they've
gotten better and the worst part is when my speech gets
slurred.

The tests have revealed that it's not any kind of growth
from the lymphoma thing (that's VERY good) and it's not a
seizure, they think it's from a combination of meds. Well, at
least lillehei does and apparently there are experts working on
the pharmacological puzzle as we speak. The jackass neurologist told me it was stress and that I should see a psychiatrist

. . . . ummmm . . . . . . don't even get me started on that guy
. . . . . he REALLY pissed me off! He will NOT be getting a
team laura t-shirt!!!!

Since these episodes have become more manageable I will
be heading back to new york tuesday, just one day late. I
couldn't be more excited. And, well, I think this year I'm
thankful for not being in the hospital on thanksgiving . . . and
being able to eat without abdominal pain and of course my
new lungs . . . I could go on and on but I think this e-mail is
long enough.

PLEASE call me if you're in new york because I've been in
and out of drug-induced states the last couple weeks and I
forget who is where and when . . . and know that every call or
e-mail or card is helping me to keep it up despite these relent-
less setbacks.

Have a happy and fun thanksgiving,

all my love always,

Laura

Subject: short update
Date: Mon, 26 Nov 2001 23:19:52 −0500
From: Laura

It was great to be in New York for almost a week. . . . . My
dad and I drove up to Boston today and I checked into the
hospital because I've been much more short of breath and having some chest pain. Well, as usual I seem to know myself well.
I have a little pneumothorax on my left side and a small pleural

effusion. We're not sure what's causing it. . . . . we'll see. . . . .
Good news is that they'll probably go ahead with the bronch
tomorrow morning. At this point I'm not sure how long I'll be in
the hospital—nice decorations, though, since I hit up kate's
paperie in new york. . . . . . . I just couldn't resist.

   hope all's well

   Laura

NOVEMBER 27, 2001

It's quiet before anyone knows I'm awake. Lie here, listen to
the wheezing, the coarse breath sounds, the rapid breaths that I
expected not to see for years. And yet this Children's Hospital is
another home. And I am sick. The future is more uncertain
than ever. At least with CF there was some kind of pattern.
Even though everyone ended up a little differently we all followed the same mold. The only one in front of me is Shawna
and she's dying. I guess the question now is how do I accept
where I am and make do and not feel like my life is inadequate?
No matter what anyone tells me I have a hard time believing
that I've done much in the last year of my life, certainly nothing compared to most my age. So I tried the transplant to get
back there, back to school. It didn't do that for me. But it has
extended my life. And the trick now is to find a purpose for
myself. Something that will keep me going. I'll let you know
when I figure something out. Then maybe I'll be able to stop
crying so much.

There's an ad for a facial exerciser to avoid facial plastic surgery. Ha.

Subject: LONG UPDATE EMAIL
Date: Wed, 05 Dec 2001 19:06:07 −0500
From: Laura

Well, here's the news . . . . . you may find it confusing but I'll
try my best to keep it as clear as possible. I don't take responsi-
bility for anything weird I say, though, because I've had some
anesthesia. . .

WHAT HAS RESULTED FROM THE CAT SCAN:

I had "the big scan" on monday to determine how my lungs
looked after the four weeks of treatment for the post transplant lymphoproliferative disease (PTLPD). Today the lymphoma
expert (her name's dr. lehman) met with the lung transplant
team and I believe the oncology fellow who has been following
my case and my father. I'll get to where I was shortly.

They have decided to do another four weeks of rituximab.
This is the monoclonal antibody I've been getting once a week
for the last four weeks. Basically, the ct scan showed that the
PTLPD has not progressed. There was some discrepancy as to
whether or not it has gotten better in the lungs, but the fact
that it has not gotten worse is a good thing and means no
chemotherapy for the time being. In fact the oncologist said for
the first time that chemo is particularly risky for lung patients

because of the bacteria that I have in my lungs and if I don't have any immune system there's more chance of getting sepsis. If you're not a doctor you may want to ignore the last sentence. GOOD NEWS: I can get some of those doses in new york at columbia at the oncology clinic like I did over thanksgiving so it's not like I'll have to be in boston christmas week or anything.

THE BIG PICTURE AS OF RIGHT NOW:

The transplant docs still think there is chronic rejection that is keeping my pfts down. They want to get the mechanical airway problems as under control as possible so that 1) I won't be having so many bronchs and 2) I won't be as out of breath and 3) they can get a better sense of how much of my pfts are suffering from the rejection. I don't know how realistic it is to think that I'll get lung function back in the 60s but you never know. We'll just have to WAIT and see . . . . . they are hoping to start me on a medication next week, an immunosuppressant called rapamycin which may help.

WHAT HAPPENED TODAY:

As some may know, I am slated to go to the spa at norwich inn tomorrow with my good friend Cynthia Butler. But the past few days I have been feeling increasingly short of breath. So, it seemed prudent not to wait until next week to have a bronch, but to have one before I go to the spa so that I'll feel as well as possible and be able to relax and rejuvenate.

Dr. Waltz left for a conference today and he usually does the dilations of the airways. So, he put into action an idea he had for quite some time. At a nearby hospital called Beth

Israel Deaconess they have a special bronchoscopy unit and a doctor who only does interventional bronchs, meaning he only does things like dilate airways and use lasers and cut out cartilage and put in stents to keep airways open. So, today I had a bronch at beth israel just to hold me over until next week when I will have another one on tuesday. Then they will do some special laser thing to try to more permanently keep the airway open. This could be the beginning of less bronchs for laura, maybe less shortness of breath. Eventually he thinks a stent in one of the airways in the left lung but right now he thinks that the right lung is what should be focused on.

Today they found that my right bronchus intermedius, which is supposed to be 12 mm wide was only 3 mm, so it's a good thing I didn't wait till next week! And, because it's an adult hospital and they were only dilating they did the procedure under conscious sedation. The first thing they did was spray what they call banana spray into my mouth, then lots of this other anesthetic stuff to get rid of my gag and cough reflex. Anyway, I barely remember the thing and I feel better now, relatively, of course, pfts still down.

THE EXCITEMENT:
So, the plan was for me to just come for the bronch and leave but I'm never that lucky. I got up to the DAY CARE UNIT and instead of recovering more, all of a sudden my oxygen saturation started to drop. It went way down. My fingertips started turning gray and my mom said I was actually looking blue. Apparently sometimes residents call them smurf kids . . . . . oh,

what a cute smurf. And the sats went down to 70 (normal
being 95–100). I was on maximum oxygen in the rebreather bag
and they were going to need me on bypap to try to get the
numbers up. The pulmonary fellow who is training with Dr. Ernst
(the bronch specialist) was great—his name's Dave.

They did an arterial blood gas and his suspicions were correct. Something called MET-HEMOGLOBIN-EMIA a VERY RARE
side effect from the drug in the banana spray they had given
me. This means that no matter how much oxygen I was on,
something was keeping the hemoglobin in my blood from bind-
ing oxygen. So they gave me this special blue medication to
reverse the side effects and in over a half hour my sats began
to improve. Except now, it's funny, my pee is blue! And
they've made me stay overnight because I may need another
dose of the med (called methaline blue) and they want to
"observe" me. So here I am at another hospital and so far so
good . . . . . nice docs, nice nurses, nice rooms. Although I do
feel like a spring chicken—everyone at the adult hospital is
OLD! DON'T GET ALARMED, EVERYTHING IS FINE NOW. . . . . .

MY SCHEDULE AS FAR AS I KNOW IT:

I will leave the hospital early tomorrow morning and go to
the spa (parents are dropping me off). Then I will return to
boston on monday december 10th, have a bronch on the
11th, maybe stay overnight at children's and have the rituximab that wednesday. I think I will stop in providence maybe
for a night or two, then head home to new york for as long as
I can. I'm sure I'll have to come back to boston for another

bronch somewhere at the end of december, but that's really too far in advance to know for sure.

LASTLY:

how am I? well, I had a rough patch for a bit, but I'm feeling better, stronger emotionally and definitely cheered up by the holiday season and the prospect of seeing lots of friends. A bit more hopeful . . . . but it's day to day and that's frustrating. Now I'm getting tired of typing and I should really put the oxygen saturation monitor back on. keep in touch and sorry again if this e-mail is too technical.

love,

Laura

DECEMBER 2001 ———————————————

I knit hats between tremors. Fold cranes between tremors. Rarely write letters by hand with tremors. Give insulin four times a day, despite tremors. Shop incessantly between 8 North Hospital stays and take pictures with my trusty Olympus to prove to those who can't be here.

Sometimes I watch movies; lately I've started to read *Harry Potter.* Yes, I have joined the masses, but proudly. The book reminds me of Roald Dahl's books when I was little. How I couldn't wait to get to the next chapter of *Matilda,* or *The Witches* or *The BFG.* Who wouldn't want a big friendly giant as a friend. Something magical in all of them, the impossible was never so, and maybe that's why I like Harry Potter now. As

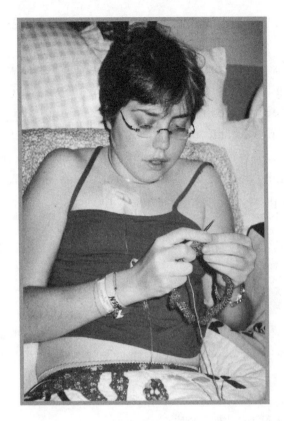

there's so much uncertainty, I like the idea of spells that can change your luck.

I plan between bronchoscopies. Two-week windows into the bustling routine of the neighborhood I'm in, the lives of the people I'm friends with. When schedules matter and time is imperative, the only thing that I focus on is when to take my medication. No more booking weeks in advance. I hope I'll make it to the spa next Thursday, but I won't know for sure until the day before. And it's been that day-to-week living all fall. Days in the hospital, though, it didn't matter—the time, the date. And suddenly it's December. And I've knit at least ten hats. And I'm still working on Will's scarf.

I've discovered that the waiting will never stop. I will always be waiting for a scan to come back, a new med to start working, a bed to be available in the hospital. Illness is not leaving my life, though I tried so hard to rid myself of it. But the waiting is the hardest part. Always wanting an answer that no one seems capable of finding because medicine just isn't there yet. Because I am a work in progress, we are learning with me.

Subject: latest news
Date: Sun, 16 Dec 2001 20:30:03 −0500
From: Laura

SO, it's been over a week since I e-mailed and I have gotten several e-mails of concern that reminded me I have not shared the news of the last week. . . . .

THE SPA AT NORWICH INN:

Lots of fun. I had just about everything you could have done—seaweed wrap, facial, normal massages, hot stone massage, manicure/pedicure. It was therapeutic and lots of fun to be with Cynthia.

I got back and had a bronch at beth israel deaconess (the adult hospital). This one was very much an "interventional bronch" meaning they did stuff that they hoped would be more permanent. Dr. Ernst (we'll just call him the lung cowboy because that's what he seems like to me!) put in a stent in my main left airway, the left bronchus. That side had remained stable for several weeks but all of a sudden it had gone down by half the size. A stent, although it increases risk of infection and may have to be changed at some point later on, should keep the airway open permanently.

They tried to do the same thing on the right side but no commercial stent would fit without blocking the airway leading to the right upper lobe (remember this blockage is in the right bronchus intermedius where three different airways meet). So, they'll have to custom-make a stent for the right side. Because of this it looks like I will require either weekly or biweekly bronchs at least until after the new year when I have plenty of time to remain in boston while they work on this airway.

GOOD NEWS:

On Thursday, before leaving Boston I went over to children's and had pfts done. It had been about a month since they were last done. And, because of all kinds of factors (LPD treatment, rejection treatment, the stent having just been put in and the airway just dilated) my pulmonary function is back in the mid-60s percentage-wise. First reaction is just utter JOY because a month ago I didn't think I'd ever get those numbers back up. Second thought is I think I will be back at school at the end of January. And third, MOST IMPORTANT THOUGHT is don't get too excited. Ups and downs. The fact that my lungs have not been damaged to the point of no return is FABULOUS, but it is possible the numbers will fluctuate. So yell thanks to the gods and then restrain yourself ☺

WHERE I AM NOW:

   Since the bronch, which was on tuesday, I had the first
dose of the second round of rituximab at the dana farber outpatient clinic (I'd forgotten how exhausted it makes me) then
I came back down to providence on thursday. I've been having
a good time here, feeling positive and seeing friends, doing
some shopping (I'm very good at what Lauren named RETAIL
THERAPY, maybe TOO good!). It's nice not to be in the middle
of exams . . . . my poor friends are agonizing over papers and
whatnot, but they've still managed to make time for me ☺
Tomorrow I will head back to boston, have my bronch on tuesday and rituximab and then down to nyc on wednesday—I
can't wait to get home. I may need another bronch at the end
of christmas week, perhaps not. If you will be in New York do
call. . . . I think I will be there for parts of january as well.

THE BIG MOVE:

   On thursday my father and I looked at an apartment downstairs in this building that has opened up. It's just a one bedroom, however I've decided to take it for the spring semester.
Basically I will never be well enough to climb these two flights
of stairs, and having that reminder every time I want to return
to my apartment doesn't help me emotionally and I think the
stairs tire me as well. No use wasting energy on those if I
don't have to. It is sad that I won't be living with abby next
semester but her friend Liz is going to move in and it's not
like I'll be very far away. Plus, Abby and I have been thinking
about getting my father to install some kind of intercom
device . . . . . hmm . . . . he likes projects! I don't know yet

what my new phone number will be for next semester but the p.o. box remains the same as does the cell number.

That's it for now. I have a TON of packing to do (for boston and trying to get my room somewhat into boxes for moving in january).

all my love,

Laura

DECEMBER 18, 2001

So I sat with Shawna tonight, for about an hour and a half. And I made dumb jokes and talked and talked and talked (she doesn't do much talking, too drugged out, too tired, too breathless) and I know that I cheered her up. I know it in my heart that it helped her to see me feeling better, to see me because I know she looks up to me. She's only sixteen.

And I got a call from Dr. Waltz and he said that he thought once all the airway problems are cleared up my PFTs could even improve—something I didn't even dream of about a month ago. He also said when asked that he didn't think I had chronic rejection anymore.

So here I sit, back on 8 North for the night, only five months out of transplant suddenly feeling like I have time again, and I'm so happy, yet I look around at Shawna and Stacy whose kidney has failed and Joselyn who is in for acute rejection and Tommy Doyle who is back and Reynaldo who has been so sick ever since I saw him for the first time this summer and . . .

1) I feel badly that I'm just passing through, and 2) I know

that I won't always pass through, that maybe even in a couple of months I'll be back where I was, and then I realize that once again I'm where I was before the transplant, that the uncertainty and unpredictability will remain for the rest of my life no matter how high or low the PFTs go. And I can live with taking pills and insulin and even more frequent bronchs to survey the lungs since I'll be on less immunosuppression than I should because of the PTLPD, but I know that it's only a matter of time before I lose out.

Not sure why, but tonight I feel the weight of all that has occurred this fall, I realize how much time I have spent in this hospital and how close I was and I just can't stop crying for myself, but also for Shawna who isn't getting better and for Jess's dad who has to have bone marrow transplant. I always wonder why I get sad when I get better. It used to frustrate my father to no end. "Why do you want to be sick?" he'd yell. After all these years I have it figured out: I think it's because I know it's not permanent. Like that fish who gets thrown back into the ocean only to get caught the next day.

DECEMBER 30, 2001 ─────────────────

Things I don't like post-transplant:

My face—puffy and ugly

Injecting insulin

Weekly bronchs

Shakiness

Extra hair on my face

Intestinal blockages and stomachaches

Don't have anything to talk about with peers—feel
lonely and useless

Maybe it'll all change in the next six months as drastically
as my life has in these past ones. It's supposed to get better . . .
keep the faith. It's hard sometimes, so hard. If I feel unhappy
with my health situation I then feel guilty—there's a donor to
be living for in addition to friends who have or are currently
dying. A month ago all I wanted was to be out of the hospital and
able to walk for blocks. I said that was enough. Now that I have
it (between bronchs) I want more—all of it. I want to be healthy.
I know, though, that
I'm asking for the
impossible. I want
to be like all of
them and I can't.
And so suddenly I
find it hard to be
around my best high
school girls. Just like
it's hard to sort of

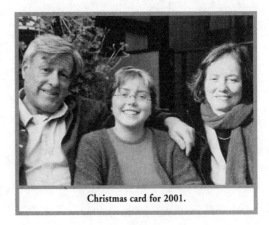

Christmas card for 2001.

have health. All or nothing is easier than gray. I spent years living in the gray area and I knew that would be the hardest possible outcome for me. I guess my New Year's resolution is to accept what I've been given and try to use my time—to be happy.

THE NEW YEAR: 2002
JANUARY 1, 2002

Tonight I feel like I'm not a fun person to be around. I take things too seriously. And I'm moody—granted I'm working on four and a half hours of sleep, I have my period, and I'm on steroids. But it's not like I walk around with a sign that says "WARNING: Has Justifiable Reasons For Not Being Someone You Want To Hang Out With." Here it is the New Year and I turn in first, leave everyone playing a fun game—and yet I can't help it. I'm tired. The responsible thing is to go to bed knowing I have to get up for nine A.M. meds and drive back to Boston. Rules and choices—I fear my next year will be dictated by them and/or hospital schedules. I flipped out today when I found out my bronch had been moved one day later—crying, crying, crying. Obviously, it's a control issue.

This next semester will be a challenge. I will be at school, still making frequent trips to the hospital, taking a few classes, staying up late, doing vital signs, taking medication—how will I focus? How will I forget about my health and still maintain it? I wish that my physical health and the meds I take to maintain it didn't affect my personality or my appearance. I'm struggling with that much more now. Perhaps today was just one of those days—but if they stack up, they could lead to the rest of my days—I will not spend them depressed. It makes me cry just thinking about the possibility. I can't tell if everyone sees how different I am now than from before the transplant. I don't like it.

I tried so hard this fall to make her days better. Found a Gumby poster on the Internet and had it sent to the hospital after she remarked how much she liked Gumby. Made a sign for her door like mine—got into a huge fight with a nurse about putting it up. Made cranes and bought other gifts—material goods to brighten her days because there was nothing I could do about what was happening to her. I knew it, she knew it. But the doctors kept saying it would get better . . . we knew they were wrong. All fall I knew it. I was surprised she lived as long as she did.

The last time I saw Shawna it was clear. She was so drugged, shaking constantly, the portable toilet set up right next to her bed. The anxiety was better—she was sleeping too much now—drugs took care of that. She lay there, expandable rings her grandmother bought on almost every finger (sometimes there's fluid buildup so fingers change size), her voice deep with lung failure, oxygen on, words used sparingly. Deep down I knew this meeting would be the last.

I said I love you. I said thank you. I said how in awe I was of her, but we didn't really get to talk because her grandmother was there. And maybe she knew it all from my eyes because I saw it in hers. And maybe she didn't need to get that letter I sent the day before her death. But how it devastated me when I realized she will never read it.

I'll never see Viglione on the patient board again. No more late-night talks, no more suited-up visits because either she or I has something the other could catch. Her death, although not unexpected, shocks my body so that I'm curled up crying.

Shawna gave me a bunny handmade at the mall. It was named Courage. Her voice is recorded, "I found this bunny and thought of you. Her name's Courage. The courage you have and the courage we share together. I hope . . ." And then it's cut off. Why didn't I ever ask what else she was going to say?

Subject: GOOD NEWS!
Date: Wed, 09 Jan 2002 22:36:31 -0500
From: Laura

I know it's been awhile since I last e-mailed . . . . no news is USUALLY good news, though, or at least that's what they used to say about kids in the hospital when I was growing up.

On December 12th as you probably know I had a stent put in my left airway to keep it open. This helped greatly and improved my pulmonary function by about 30%. I continued to have weekly bronchs. Last friday, after a delay when fed-ex didn't deliver the Iowa custom-made stent on time (just my luck), they put the new stent on the right side (the airway that was closing down every week) in addition to a topical agent that kills the overgrowth of cells. Today I had pfts and . . . . my pulmonary function is back up to 92%!!!!! This is FABULOUS news. Now we just have to hope that they stay there. I also had a ct scan today to determine what will come next in terms of PTLPD treatment—maybe more rituximab, maybe not. Not clear when I will find out those results.

My schedule for the next couple weeks: I will have a bronch tomorrow so they can have a look, maybe apply some more cell-killing cream, we'll see. I'll be in new york from friday to sunday, then I'm flying to visit a friend in Ohio for about five days. Then another couple days in new york before I head back to brown probably around the 20th of january. Classes start on January 23rd. I hope to take 3, one writing class and probably a couple political science classes, but we'll see.

I have a bit of a sinus infection, but other than that I'm feeling pretty well and hoping that will last. Hope that you had a good new year—I was in Vermont with friends from high school, which was a lot of fun.

all my love,

Laura

JANUARY 16, 2002, DOG LIFE ───────

The leash has been extended, I'm in Ohio. I just flew into Cleveland to visit my close friend Will, at Oberlin College. Now it's not a short, set length, but one that allows me to travel. Cut me more slack, but just as easily take it away from me. I stand as the winter-worn trees in Oberlin, reflected in the parking lot's puddle of melted snow. Although surrounded by others, each grows alone, branches never able to merge into one.

Subject: january health news

Date: Sat, 19 Jan 2002 12:19:43 -0500

From: Laura

hey guys

Here's the health update . . . sorry it's been awhile but I just got back from ohio—it was GREAT to get away from the east coast and spend time with my friend.

My last bronch was SHORT and went very well. They said all stents in place, all airways looked good. So hopefully that'll be my last time at the BI (adult hospital)—they were starting to know and like me, though, so I think I'll be safe if I ever have to go back there for stent repairs, etc. . . . hee hee. I will have to have semi-regular bronchs done to monitor for rejection, but more on a monthly or bi-monthly basis.

GOOD NEWS: the ct scan showed NO new nodules, so no more rituximab for now. In terms of the PTLPD, I'll probably be having ct scans once a month for a while to keep an eye out for recurrence. Unfortunately, the ct scan also showed some new big infiltrate in the right upper lobe and one in the lower left, I think. So, I'm taking an oral antibiotic for my sinus infection and Vancomycin by IV for the pneumonia. I should be on the Vanco for several weeks at least. I've been coughing a lot, a bit tired, but not such a big deal since it's a treatable bacterial infection as opposed to a fungus or something like that.

And tomorrow I head back to Brown to try again. I'm going to try to cut down the number of health updates because hopefully there won't be much to update about if all goes well. Whenever you want to know, though, just send an e-mail and ask or do so in person. And in about two weeks I'll be 21—weird.

I've been pretty down lately, and still trying to deal with Shawna's death (it was one week ago today, she was 16, had chronic rejection) I think it's going to ache for a while. but I guess that's all part of the process in addition to this constant uncertainty I'm faced with.

It's supposed to snow today—can't wait! Let me know if/when you're back in town for those that will be around this semester. And for those who aren't, keep me updated on all escapades!

all my love,

Laura

JANUARY 31, 2002 ————————————————

Tomorrow is February, the first day of which would be my grandfather's 93rd birthday. First his, then the groundhog's shadow, then me. The Russian twins Aunt Judy almost adopted were born on February 2nd. But Vera and Nadya have a July birthday—like Uncle Jim.

After a few days back at Brown, I'm back in. It's been awhile since an admission. I hope this will be short. Two nights is nothing. But it's a trip back to this world of sick struggle to get just that much better. Both Joselyn and Michelle are on the floor now and Reynaldo. A liver and two kidneys respectively. Jos has attitude. Last night, being escorted from the playroom to take meds in her Disney nightgown the five-year-old states, "Don't touch me, just don't touch me"—overdramatic sigh—"mothers!" Apparently one time when an IV nurse came to put in an IV she said in the rudest tone possible, "You are the ugliest thing I've ever seen." If I was that small I'd use words as weapons, too. What a smart girl. She's facing rejection, or rather, her mother, Josie, is.

Mom arrived on the train last night, her flight attendant–style luggage in tow. Abby was here from Providence taking over my knitting when I saw her through the glass and its sign painted by Jackie—a get-well-soon heart to all the "kidz" on 8 North. Yesterday was fever and coughing and vomiting. First after PFTs in the bathroom, then in clinic—the trash can. Once I half-missed— I don't think it's too noticeable on my shoe, no odor at least. Low blood pressure, weight loss. "How do you feel about coming in?"

"I just want to lie down."

CT scan showed only improvement, and so I'm put on the add-on schedule for the OR. Today I waited from eight in the morning, when I was woken up during rounds, until three. Got back from recovery around six.

FEBRUARY 3, 2002, 12:21 A.M. ———

It's that day I used to revere. The one I would mark on any calendar I found, whether actually belonging to a friend or a stranger. February was the greatest month in the world, the third the greatest day, and 1981 the greatest year to be born. And today, twenty-one years later I sit in Providence, Rhode Island, in boxers and a T-shirt, by myself, not sure how to react. Alone is okay. I don't think anyone knows what to say. Pure happiness, while expected by most, is not it. Too simple. My fingernails are blood red, three of them garnished with rhinestone flowers.

Friday night I was on roller skates, in a small rink in Warwick where the seven of us one-timers stuck out. Nothing mattered to me. Around I go, and the feet remember—birthday parties on Wollman Rink's concrete, ice-skating lessons at Rockefeller Center with Melanie. I used to cross over on each turn, right over left, glide. Calculate how to control the skates, glide. My hair just fits into a ponytail, a tiny one, I have big hoops in my ears, a tight shirt, and unfocused eyes (I'm not quite good enough to close them). I can go anywhere on these skates. I speed up, move quickly past Kat, use leg muscles I'd forgotten were there; I don't cough. Around and around with the exercise breeze—something I've missed on foot and only found when I drive my car. But now the breeze and the sweat and the gliding and that recognition—of health. Free for tonight, for tomorrow; I miraculously forget to wonder about next week.

Now I sit, crowded by books about Congress and public policy and doctors and the stress that results from being behind in all my reading. "You're taking four classes?" is the general reaction. A confident "yes" or a hesitant "for now" is my usual response. Tonight I marvel at what has changed in my last year and wish that in the upcoming months I can try it all again—those things that became scary reminders—the ones I haven't even considered doing since I was twelve. I want to. I'm not going to sit and worry—enough. It's my goal, a birthday resolution. A year from now I want to look back and feel proud of myself. To know "Laura" again, and know that the medical textbook's back on the shelf.

JAVIER ——————————————————————

How's Jav doing? Like, HA, but with a V at the end: HA-V. I would call him that for short in later years, sort of to make fun, to make sure it was clear I knew he wasn't such a tough guy. I think I got it from Genevieve or Rechelle, maybe Kristal, child-life specialists at the hospital.

I said it today at brunch just like any other, just like many others.

"How's Jav doing?"

"You haven't heard?"

That's enough, I don't need to ask but I go through the formalities. "Oh no. When did he die?"

"I'm sorry, I thought you would have heard by now."

Just like I said to Daniella Michilli in Dr. Ores's Park Avenue office. Daniella escaped death by transplant just before Christmas later that year. I wonder if she's still alive. I doubt I'd recognize her. She asked about Gina that morning. "I just came from her funeral," I said.

The older girl was shocked. "When did she die?"

Always ask when; it seems as if knowing where I was when he died leads me to believe I felt something missing. Was I thinking about him that day? Or do I tell myself that to feel better because I hadn't talked to him since the end of December?

Javier. I was twelve when I met him; he was one of the CF crew. They were the cool hospital gang, always sneaking here or there, getting restless. Miguel, the leader, died before I ever got to know him. He was a staff favorite. The hospital was silent for the rest of that August. It was never the same.

And Damien I barely talked to. The social worker Winsome talked about him, though, years later, reminding me that I should take advantage of my Make-a-Wish; Damien had been too sick when he finally decided to fulfill his dream—hiking in the West. Instead he met one of the Mets, I think. Apparently Boomer Esiason, even though he had a newborn with CF, wouldn't meet Damien. I saw Boomer touring the hospital once with one of the pulmonary attendings, Dr. Quittel. I got on the elevator down from tea (every Wednesday on the eleventh floor) and he was there—blond and big. Down to the eighth floor and I ran into 838.

"Nikky, I just saw Boomer Esiason in the elevator!"

"Did you get his autograph?"

"No, I didn't think of it." I was a failure. That autograph could've cheered Nikky. He had diabetes from the steroids. Nikky Cooley. He kept trying to dye his hair purple, was only a year older than I when he died a couple months after Damien. I had a crush on him.

Talmisha. She died that year, too, on New Year's Eve day. The first of four straight years I would ring in the New Year in the hospital. She was dying. I knew it. Bypap, linguini limbs, fevers. I went in every day to see her. Maybe I could cheer her up, I thought. She seemed to be happy to see me, or she pretended. She told me how they kept saying she would recover.

Zeke, the North Jersey kid who had a mysterious twin but didn't have to check his sugars because he knew how much insulin to give himself—he always made us laugh. One night he came into my room with a contraption. He'd taken apart three hospital phones and made a three-way calling system.

Talmisha didn't know that I was listening when he called her room.

"This is different," she confided in him. "It's not right. They keep drawing blood. I am scared." "Scared" meant death to me. CF patients are never scared, until they approach the unknown.

Lee, an intern I liked, came into my room. She struck up regular conversation. And then in the middle she told me. "Laura, Talmisha just died." I burst into tears; we took a walk down the hallway, off the unit, to the dead of the hospital on a major holiday. Later I visited the nurses' station. Cathy, the nurse who sang songs, had tears in her eyes.

Years later I heard about Talmisha's older sister who'd had CF and Miguel's older sister Loren who'd had CF. And there was a girl named Laura Smith, who'd had CF. Legends in rooms I now frequented. Javier'd known all of them.

One time he came in coughing up blood. I stood by his sink the next morning as the red paint poured out. I got the nurse. What did it mean? Would that happen to me? I never asked him. He had a laugh that shook his whole body—like most of us it turned into a cough. He dumped water over Ginny at July Fourth picnics. He was admitted once when a girlfriend smashed a glass bowl and a piece of it got into his toe. There was some fight at the playroom—the girl sort of beat him up, his port needle came out, security was called. Most stories involving him made me laugh. Javier got a tattoo of a boy giving the finger on one of his biceps. For the longest time Dr. Ores didn't know about it. One day she saw it, laughed, and patted him on the head. He did a funny impersonation of her. "This is Celia Orrrrressss." Cough, cough, cough. Javier was married when he died.

I wonder if he was scared. Genevieve said he'd declared about his decision not to have a lung transplant, "I came into this world with CF, I'm going out of it with CF."

Braver than I'll ever be.

8 NORTH

The Solid Organ Transplant Unit. Authorized Personnel Only marks all doors that enter into our part of the eighth floor. This is to prevent patients with low immune systems from being exposed to unnecessary germs. More peaceful on the surface than most floors I've spent time on. Small unit—only eight beds. You're a kidney, a liver, a small bowel, or lungs. Hearts have their own floor. A mix of new and old—you come to this floor right after the transplant and you hope you never come back.

At night, once Zelda the desk clerk leaves, the phone rings until one of two nurses can get to it. In the day it's a woman named Shawna who calls out names of fellows responding to pages. The past couple evenings a "broken" sign has been stuck with tape on the door of the tub room. This is the only way to keep people out after Sophie has cleaned it for me. A public bathroom has a bath that I actually like? Well, that's why it's cleaned before I use it. But the bath is comfortable.

Even in my sickest moments this fall I would try to make it to the hot water. Cleanse myself, immerse in bubbles, maybe wash my hair. When I was too tired to stand up, leaning my head back was enough. After years of washing my own hair in the sink with gold medal speed, this bath trick has come in handy, too.

Sometimes friends would assist me, which basically meant making sure I didn't topple over stepping in. Or my mom. She runs the bath like no other—just the right temperature. Beeping echoes, there go some clogs, an announcement overhead, "So and so please return to 10 East. So and so please return to 10 East." I was on that floor before the transplant. But those noises are distant when I'm in the tub.

And I realize it's about baths and toilets. That's how I know I'm home. The apartment in New York, the tenth floor there, the apartment in Brookline, the hospital in Boston, my apartment now in Providence. But in the dorms, I was never home—no sense of permanence or privacy. I could search out a bathroom maybe down in the depths of my freshman dorm, next to the boiler and the overflowing cans of empty beer. But it wasn't mine. I didn't know it. It doesn't matter which room on 10 South or 8 North, it's all the same feeling. Besides, I've been in all of them by now anyway.

Subject: health stuff
Date: Wed, 20 Feb 2002 22:07:26 −0500
From: Laura

bad news.

I am once again in the hospital. I came in on Monday night after being in new york for a brief two days (and not feeling that great). I woke up that morning with a fever and coughing a ton and so I ended up in the Boston ER. Today I had a bronch to look for why I have a new infiltrate in the right lung

and I had an endoscopy (basically doing biopsies in the esophagus and tummy) to look for worsening reflux. And there's
something up with my red blood cells. . . . they just keep
going low (significant anemia).

We won't get culture and biopsy results for a few days,
BUT they did find in the bronch that my right stent has slid
down and is blocking part of the entrance into my right middle
lobe where the new pneumonia was found.

Another bronch has been set for friday (yup, two days from
now). It will be done at the BI and then I'll be transferred back
here. I think I may be here for a few days until they get everything sorted out—what is causing what, etc. I'm on two new
antibiotics also and so I'm already feeling a little better. I was
back in school, although not feeling great, so I'd love to get
whatever's going on taken care of.

keep in touch
Laura

Subject: long day!
Date: Fri, 22 Feb 2002 22:50:00 −0500
From: Laura
To: A friend

had bronch number two today—turns out the stent hadn't
moved, just some wires sticking down, so that wasn't causing the pneumonia. In fact the stent itself, on the right, is
very much in place with tissue growing around it, etc. I knew
I would've had more of a sense of shortness of breath if it

had moved. But I wasn't going to argue with what they said they saw.

My doctor's away this week, but back monday so things like chronic anémia and reflux and home iv will be discussed then. I was super discouraged today, though. Transferred by ambulance to the BI and back and lots of waiting and I was hungry and moody because of that whole diabetes thing with not eating . . . . . . I'm getting frustrated.

Today I watched it. Granted, anesthesia and swollen throat from the rigid bronch doesn't help the general mood, nor does waiting for an hour and a half to get transferred across the street! And starting to get worried that this is the beginning of another hospital season, just different problems. And with Shawna gone, and Javier passing away, and Joselyn, this little girl who got a liver a month after I did, not doing well . . . . it's a lot. Sometimes it seems like too much. And I find myself just asking for drugs—can't they give me more benadryl so I can jut sleep until the bronch? Or last night I couldn't fall asleep—can't I just have more trazedone? I used to hate sleeping medication, or say I wouldn't take it because, well, I never needed it and now I'm just begging. My tolerance is definitely growing and that only makes it harder.

those are tonight's thoughts

Laura

Subject: My last few days
Date: Thu, 28 Feb 2002 18:11:27 −0500
From: Laura
To: A friend

yes, my last pfts
were 102%, so
that's good news.
Hopefully they'll
stay there for once!
I don't think I've
had the same pfts
two weeks straight
yet . . . . I knew
I was sick with that
dumb 92, hee hee,

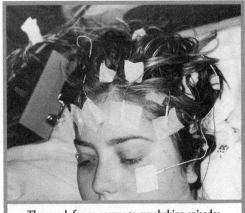

The search for an answer to my shaking episodes.

never thought I'd be saying that!

Unfortunately the anxiety is awful. Still having panic
attacks. I've talked to dr. burr more in the last few days than
I had all fall from out of the hospital. Anyway, starting me on
something more long-acting than ativan, you take it just
twice a day, starts with a c and it's a benzo. I'm dropping or
maybe switching to auditing my hardest class—the one on
congress. Pretty down about that, but I have to. At least
right now there's no way I can make it through the semester
with the amount of work I have and I can't even do the work
well, which is a shame. So of course I'm feeling a bit like a
failure with the anxiety, and the taking less classes, but I
know it's what I have to do. My mom is here with me in providence for a few days until we break the cycle that STARTED

because they refused to give me IV ativan when I had the first one—that bad resident . . . . . I better not have her again!

Laura

Subject: Re: health stuff
Date: Sat, 02 Mar 2002 21:37:53 −0500
From: Laura
To: A friend

Got out of the hospital last tuesday, still doing six iv doses at home, but feeling SO much better I can't even tell you. Not all phlegmy like I was before and the appetite is finally back. About time—I'm down to110 pounds! It's been sort of hard since I got out of the hospital—anxiety attacks still for the first couple of days. Now I'm on a new medication (clonazepam or something instead of ativan) and it's helping with those, although we're in the process of switching my antidepressant, which means tapering for a while so I feel overly emotional.

I'm not able to handle when I don't have plans at the moment, like waiting to figure out what I may do tonight. I'm unable to really concentrate when I'm alone—basically I'm depressed. But it's all just a part of the process I think. I guess I can't ignore whatever it is I'm feeling deep down—I'm just too exhausted to deal in some ways. All the waiting and the uncertainty of the past seven and a half months have gotten me to this point. It makes me sad, to think of what possibility there is, that I'm unable to really use it at the moment.

But eventually I'll get through this, too. It was so bad that my mom came up from nyc and she's still here. Finally tonight staying at a hotel instead of in my apartment. Hopefully I can get through the next couple of nights . . . part of what's hard is that it's midterms so most people are studying hard and I should be too but I just want to get my mind off it all. I had a lot of fun last night, though. I'm sure I'll pick myself up and go somewhere tonight.

sorry to ramble on, sometimes it just happens when you start typing.

hope all's well . . .

Laura

EMOTIONAL VIBRATIONS

It began in November, although I didn't believe the neurologist then. He said the strange and uncontrollable shaking was from stress. "Do you see a psychiatrist?" I found his tone accusatory. Of course I can handle it all, why would my body be physically reacting to emotions? But all the neurology tests were done: head CT, MRI of my head, and two EEG tests—they glue about twenty-eight electrodes onto your head and monitor the brain waves during episodes. I was a sight. At the time the ruling by all but this one neurologist was that the shaking was from a combination of all the medications I was taking. A pharmacological puzzle. However, it was never solved; small doses of Ativan were helping and other medical issues took the forefront. Looking back, I know it was the first time my emotions tried to break through my stoic wall. They (hospital staff) all thought I was handling it so well.

I'm in the Bronx on the corner of East 174th and Westminster Avenue, heading back to Brown from my grand-mother's house in Riverdale. The Sunoco station was the first place I pulled into for directions. Instead of taking my usual route—the Bruckner Expressway to the Deegan to 95, I take the Madison Avenue Bridge to the Cross Bronx Expressway and get flustered, doubting my ability to navigate the elevated highways that weave through New York City's boroughs.

Stop next to a pump, unbuckle the seat belt, lock the door, and jog into the food mart to ask the man for directions. He points to written directions to 95—perhaps many get lost this way. Run to the car, ready to get back to the road, my mix tape, thoughts about my weekend at home in New York. And then I see what I have done—the key is locked in the car.

A man at a nearby pump says he has plenty of friends in the neighborhood that could open the car. He'll bring one back. Thirty minutes later I give up waiting. Walk to the nearby pay phone, and call AAA. A locksmith will arrive in an hour.

So I make more phone calls to memorized numbers. Mom wants to know what part of the Bronx I'm in. "Oh, lovely," is her reply. I return to the car, watch all the livery cab drivers pull in to fill up, and it starts. My right arm shakes. A small tremor, then more. My right leg begins shaking, both legs. A stranger thinks I'm cold. "Yeah, coat's locked in the car, too." But I know. I know it's an attack, that if it escalates I could end up in some hospital.

That makes me worry more, the fear of medical personnel who don't know my history taking care of me. I start telling myself in my head: "You can do it. This will work out. You're stronger than this. Don't be afraid." A self-motivation, anti-attack chant. Relax, relax, it'll be fine. Walk around, make a couple more calls, my hands shake so much that it's hard to dial the numbers. Finally, time passes, and I win. I overcome the fear. It's the first time I've done it. I talk to the Russian man behind the glass who tells me how if he's not careful and people steal gas it gets taken out of his salary. How his English, even after three years in New York, "not so good. But children, they good."

The locksmith shows how easy it is to break into my car with the proper equipment—luckily my dad has dented the car over the years so it's not all that appealing to steal. I sign some paper, my hand still trembling a bit, and find my way back to 95, and driving.

CAUTION: SPEED BUMPS AHEAD

I found the road sign in an antique store in Manchester, Vermont, the day before the New Year. Had to buy it. The current definition of my life. Each bump small enough to slow down the car, sometimes bring it almost to a halt, but not big enough to stop it completely. That's what this anxiety is—a series of speed bumps. I don't see them as warnings, but obstacles, small ones. Each attack, another attempt by fear to take over. Each recovery, the car plops down on the other side of the bump. The hope: to find a road without any speed bumps.

IN MY HEAD ————————————————————————

I don't really know why the anxiety attacks started. I think the hospital is just a stressful place for me to be now. I have a lot of traumatic memories from this past autumn, and whenever something medical is uncertain I seem to be unable to handle it—like, for example, extended waiting for medical procedures. I guess I'm just worn out. But the truth is it doesn't have much to do with me. I don't choose to start shaking, to cry, to get upset about my life. In fact, I carry a lot of guilt each day, for my two younger friends who died this fall (post-transplant) and all those other friends. If I've gone through all this, made it this far, especially after November when I was facing death once again, and they weren't lucky enough, I don't understand why I can't just accept where I am and be content.

Why should I be upset that just about every food I really like gives me reflux? Why should I be upset that I just spent two months on IV antibiotics? It's no different from before. All I could hope for three months ago was to stay alive. But now I just want more, one always does. All of it has piled up and now I have to release. That's what the shaking is. Perhaps there's even a certain amount of shaking that must go on for my body to accept what it is now, to reach that point where change is positive.

It's Sunday night; the census on the transplant floor is low enough that they have only one nurse. He's a paternalistic man with a heavy Boston accent. I joke with him about his "cah" and his "watah." I take my normal sleeping medication (2 mg of

Ativan and 50 mg of Trazedone). But about twenty minutes later my right arm begins shaking. It starts small, but becomes increasingly violent. He responds to the call bell. "I need more Ativan to stop this shaking."

"Kiddo, you just had some, there's no way you're getting more. You won't keep breathing."

Okay. He's the nurse. But it doesn't get better. I ring again and request to see the resident on call. She won't come down to see me until after several pulmonary admissions. The shaking has increased now—my head, one leg, probably, and I'm sobbing uncontrollably. "I need help, why won't anyone listen to me?"

Phone my father; he comes over to the hospital and threatens to page the pulmonary attending on call himself if I'm not given more Ativan. Not even IV, they give it to me by mouth—which takes forty-five minutes to kick in. The shaking continues, the crying continues. "I need something now!" No one but my father gives a damn. Perhaps even he doesn't understand the relief I'm craving. I am physically unable to control my body's emotional reactions, the shaking perhaps a way of getting it all out, all that anger and frustration and fear.

Dr. Burr, my psychiatrist, is upset. The next morning she tells me the worst thing that can be done for an anxiety attack is to prolong it—exactly what was done that night.

Another attack that evening. I can't sit still, I feel uncomfortable, and the shaking pains my body, like a long workout; my upper arms ache, but I can't just call it a day. This night, however, both parents are here. Camilla's my nurse and it's a different resident. He, instead of being influenced by what a more experienced nurse says, calls Dr. Burr, and she says he should give IV

Ativan. When it kicks in I begin to feel myself again, able to relax, to sink into a bed as one does on a cold night. I feel safe. Not that I'm afraid an attack will cause me to die, but rather that it will cause me to lose myself.

I am a witness to an "incident" on campus. Blatant racial profiling of a black student, the police tackling him to the ground all because he refuses to show his Brown ID. There he sits, handcuffed, in the dirt next to one of the oldest buildings on campus, yelling, "Why do I have to show my ID? What about everyone else around here? It's because I'm black. This is bullshit!" All he did was walk across campus. After he and his friend are taken by the police the shaking starts.

A friend, Hentyle, walks around the corner. I start crying to him, left arm shaking, left leg shaking. I tell the dean of student life on the scene how horrific it was. And I believe it was horrific. I know it goes on every day, but watching someone else losing control reminds me of my own loss. I can't stop the shaking. The concern in Hentyle's eyes grows; he and some others sit me down. And now my whole body is shaking, asking, "Why?" Why him, why me, why anyone? I feel dizzy, stare farther and farther from the close friends who keep talking. A dean is afraid of what he sees, calls EMS.

But the fear grows deeper when EMS arrives. They don't know my medical history, they don't understand. Even expert physicians get confused. I don't want to go to the hospital. I just want it to stop. I refuse to go until someone from Boston is contacted. Cry a bit out of frustration. No hospital, please, no. It's the shaking that dominates, though, not hysteria. On the Brown Daily Jolt (an anonymous Internet forum) they refer to me as "the quivering girl."

Abby rides in the ambulance. The sirens. I smile. She says I look like some kind of devil, maybe a cat plotting to steal the steak from the table. I like the sirens. We arrive at the hospital and I keep saying, "That's not what you say to someone with a panic disorder. That's not what you say to someone with a panic disorder." Then, "I need to see a doctor, making me wait is not what should be done for a panic attack! Stop asking questions, that's not what you do for someone with a panic disorder. I need Ativan. Give me Ativan." Been bossy since birth.

Have I become a drug addict?

The shot goes into my right arm. Ow. But then, relief. After twenty minutes the marathon is over, the shaking has calmed down. Hentyle and Abby and Hannah and Nyla and Chris rotate. Hentyle and Abby bring me home. It was the shortest ER visit ever. Until Monday night. It begins again. I call Ali, ask her to come over and she can tell in my voice what's happening. She arrives unsure how to help. We try me on the bed, her stroking my back, but it doesn't do it. Finally I agree to go to the hospital. We pick up her sister Brooke and head to Hasbro again, the local children's hospital. The shaking is uncontrollable, mainly from the shoulders through the arms, my head a bit. Once I'm lying on the stretcher my right leg kicks in, too. I get the Ativan and gradually relax, although it's not as fast this time. The physician asks, "Your PFTs are so good. What is there to be anxious about?" At the moment I take it as an insult, feel I have to justify why. We all did—Abby has arrived by this point. She was in class when the attack happened.

Now, a couple weeks later, I see he was trying to help. Trying to show me a different way to look at where I am. I'm trying to get there, trying, trying.

First day of spring, but there's snow. A normal clinic visit. Bloodwork, PFTs, an X ray. PFTs are down about 8 percent, but who can complain about 99 percent? Then I head to Fegan 5, sit in room 7 this time. And the talk ensues. I've lost five pounds in two weeks—why? Reflux, sinus infection, anxiety/depression, stomachaches, high blood sugars means peeing out calories. It's multi-factorial, we like to say in the medical world. And all I can see is the weight continuing to plummet, me in a size zero instead of a now slightly roomy size 2, getting another lung infection and unable to fight it. All I can see is Shawna at the end, her thin body so weak—if only her nutrition had been better, we all said. And here I see mine going down and I want, I believe I need, help.

A button is a feeding tube. I used to have one. I used to hate it. It feels more foreign in a body than a central line under the skin. Even more foreign than lungs that aren't yours. "We've never had a patient ask for one before." What does that mean? Am I just so wrapped up in the anxiety that I can't think clearly anymore? No. I deeply feel a need. And to wait until I'm another ten pounds less seems absurd to me. Waiting is old now. Let's do it, let's be proactive, let's make me well, please.

Subject: update
Date: Sun, 31 Mar 2002 18:07:05 –0500
From: Laura
To: Chapin pals

here's the latest

had a successful pedialyte feeding two nights ago, then last night with the real stuff went ok . . . . . . but I finally pooped today so hopefully tonight's will be much better and I won't have such a tummy ache. The panic attacks, now that I've had the triple surgery have calmed down (sinuses—polyp removal, cleanout, button, bronch with NEGATIVE biopsies for rejection! yeah, now the pred's down to 10). The panic attacks are the worst in the hospital I think because there's a post-trauma aspect to them. Dr. Burr's away this week but dr. beesley's been covering—she's great, I really like her, too. How has your week/end gone/been going?

I'll be in the hospital probably just until tomorrow (cross those fingers!) then back to providence and school. Saw good ol' dr. brown (he's done all my interventional radiology stuff) in the cafeteria and he stopped to hear the latest news. I like docs that keep up even when they aren't currently involved. Yesterday morning dr. lillehei (my surgeon) said his teenagers were still asleep at home and I said it wasn't fair, that he should get them up (this was at 8:30) and he said I like to pick my battles and I felt like saying, "me too." Because it was a battle to get this g-tube placed then nutrition came in and did the percentile and suddenly everyone realized just how underweight I really was. Figures.

And this morning my parents and I had a little smoked

salmon easter brunch . . . . so happy easter to those who celebrate it and happy belated passover REBECCA especially!
Sorry there wasn't any funny matzoh card this year I
keep trying to get better. Watching star wars yesterday and
you know what yoda, whose poster is hanging up behind my
bed, says? Luke Skywalker goes "All right, I'll give it a try."
And Yoda goes "NO! Try not. Do or not do, there is no try."

ob-la-di-ob-la-da, life goes on, rah, la la la la life goes
on. . . . .

love you,

Laura

A.M. ROUTINE

"Morning," says the latest CD in the dream machine alarm
clock. It was a gift from several friends for my twenty-first birthday. Lie in the pillow stack, look at the ceiling, some of the pictures on the wall, find motivation. Sit up.

Read the numbers on the feeding pump. Last night I went at
a rate of 70, I got 700 ccs in. I'm making progress. That's about
three cans of formula. It's only been a few weeks since the placement of the feeding tube in my stomach. Getting up to the rate
nutrition wants will take time. Turn off the pump. Doing the
"feeds" as they're called when I'm awake makes me want to vomit.
I'm full in the mornings so I don't eat breakfast. After all, I did
get 1,300 calories while asleep. You'd think my digestive tract
would want another nap.

Take five enzymes for the feeding I did overnight. Swallow.

They're the ones I take every time I eat—half yellow, half gray. Called Ultrase MT20. They digest because my pancreas doesn't. I take five before the feeding starts, too.

VITAL SIGNS come first. I have a binder that Louella decorated in August. Blood pressure gets done with the automatic blood pressure machine. Press Start and it inflates, then starts dropping. Try to do the temperature at the same time. Mark down results in the book. It's my home chart.

Check my blood sugar—click, prick, encourage a drop of blood from my finger, the Accu-check strip sucks blood up like the vampire it is. Wait forty long seconds for a reading. Mark it down.

Put my finger in the painless pulse/ox. It beeps to the rate of my heart, tells me what my oxygen saturation is. Mark down those results.

Lastly, I do my home spirometry. A gadget that I blow into as hard as possible for as long as possible and it tells me how many liters of air is in the first second that I blow out—it's a home pulmonary function test. Of course, not as accurate as the million-dollar one in the hospital, but it's a way for me to monitor lung function at home. As long as it's in the same range as days before I know I don't have some acute rejection. Mark those readings down.

Mark down any complaints I can think of—in each clinic visit the nurse coordinator or Dr. Waltz will look through the book. Close it, I'm done. Put it in one of two drawers my father and his friends built. They slide out from under the bed and I keep all my equipment in one, all my extra pill bottles in the other.

9 A.M. IS PILL TIME. At night it's 9 P.M. On the transplant floor that's when nurses are busiest. All their patients need pills at the same time. I have one of those pill organizers at home that most elderly own. I fill it once a week, as if I'm playing Mancala again in third grade, an African stone game we all fought over at recess.

Cellcept. T-cell inhibitor. Pale grayish purple. Actually says what it is and the dosage on it—most don't. Swallow.

Four tiny coated pills: FK506. They're small, but they powerfully protect me—the main immunosuppressant. Swallow them together.

They cause high blood pressure, so I take the dark pink Procardia XL. (When I was first out of transplant I needed twice as much Procardia and another blood pressure med called enalapril.) Swallow.

Then the prednisone. It's the third immunosuppressant in the cocktail. Right after transplant I took 50 milligrams every morning. Now I'm down to 10—just one white pill that says DAN on its flat top and bottom. When I was on more my face puffed up like a chipmunk. I still shudder when I see those pictures from the fall, even though most told me it wasn't so bad. Swallow.

Nexium, "the new purple pill," as it's advertised on TV, helps with the reflux. I used to take Prilosec twice a day, but now just one of these in the morning. Swallow.

Ursodiol, a pink and white-coated capsule helps the liver function better. Took it before the transplant, too. Swallow.

Celexa. Tries to keep me happy. One of those—white, not coated. Swallow.

Green pill is clonazepam—it's sort of like a tranquilizer. Prevents the horrible anxiety attacks. Swallow.

And added just a couple days ago—Clarinex, for allergies, light blue. Swallow.

Vitamins, too. People with CF don't absorb the fat soluble ones as well: that's A, D, E, and K. One multivitamin, small and red. Swallow.

Tiny yellow uncoated vitamin K. It's round. Swallow.

Vitamin E is a football-shaped yellowish fluid-filled pill. Swallow.

The wart pill is iron. Black, oddly round. Swallow.

Monday, Wednesday, and Friday I take Bactrim, an uncoated, big-sized antibiotic—it's prophylactic treatment. I used to take Acyclovir every day—an antiviral, but I'm off that now that I'm nine months out. Swallow.

Done with pills. Close the morning part of the daily pill organizer, put the container back in row with the others for the week. Flonase nasal spray next—two squirts in each nostril. It tastes like flowers smell.

When I decide to do it, the Nystatin swish and swallow comes here. It's yellow, doesn't taste great, but prevents fungus from growing in your mouth and throat—no cold sores. If it fit in the pill container I'd take it every day, four times a day, like I'm supposed to. But it's harder to pour something out in addition.

Now the insulin injection, if I remember at this point. Sometimes I don't do it until I'm already dressed. Usually pick the legs or the tummy, but now there isn't much fat anywhere, so it hurts more. Alcohol-swab the glargine vial—it's a new twenty-four-hour insulin, as opposed to NPH which lasts for twelve hours, or Humalog which peaks within minutes. Draw up eight units with my thin syringe. Alcohol the injection site; today it's my tummy. Pinch the site with the left hand. Inject with the right. Push in the insulin. Release left hand. Pull needle out. Put it in the infectious sharps container.

At this point I take the feeding bag and tube and wash them out in the kitchen sink, make sure the formula cans have been put in recycling, make sure that I don't smell like Nutren. Sometimes I shower, sometimes I don't. Put on an outfit. Sometimes I try to look coordinated, but if I have a class I'm rushing to that doesn't always happen. Gather books together, my wallet, my cell phone, my keys. Walk the two blocks to the main green and try to blend in with all the other college students I pass.

APRIL 22, 2002

I just returned from the supermarket. I carried the bags in myself. I put away the groceries. I did the remaining dishes in the sink. Now there's reading for class tomorrow that I just don't feel like doing.

April 15th was my nine-month transplant anniversary. I spent the evening with a close friend. Each month I remember the 15th. Most others, including my parents, have to be coaxed to remember the significance. For me, though, April was different from previous months.

Finally, after a couple months of shaking, my psychiatrist

realized that perhaps one of my medications was adding to the problem. And sure enough, there it was—Reglan. It can cause Parkinsonian-like shaking, severe depression, anxiety, and even restlessness. A week off the medication and I am more myself. This month, for the first time, I felt well on my anniversary.

Nine months later I realize I'm still standing. In fact, I'm the tallest I've been since the transplant. I played Frisbee the other day on the main green. I played kickball the other night. I'm beginning to see some kind of future for myself, to let hope seep back into my vocabulary. Perhaps I have finally reached that mythical plateau.

Still, though, I don't have an appetite. Just doing the overnight feedings and hoping that those are enough to keep my weight up. I wish I were hungry. Didn't even have dinner tonight.

And since December a wart has been growing on my left toe. I'd never had one before, but without T-cells to fight viruses I'm prone. It's the only thing Brown Health Services can really treat me for—all the other medical stuff is too specialized. He picks at it with a razor blade, my foot shakes because of my baseline tremor, then he freezes it off. But it keeps coming back. This stupid wart. I've been to the clinic at least five times.

Now there's another small one, lower down on the same toe. The initial wart still grows in a viral clump. If it isn't plummeting lung function or a partially blocked bowel, it's a wart or allergies. Sometimes it's all four. But it keeps coming back, despite modern medicine. This stupid wart. It keeps coming back.

So I relish the freedom I have at the moment and try desperately to appreciate it. Listening to upbeat music like Madonna's *Immaculate Collection* helps. Even harder is not worrying about what else, like the stupid wart, will return. The goal is to be vigilant without letting my health rule my life. I'm ready, so ready, to reach that place.

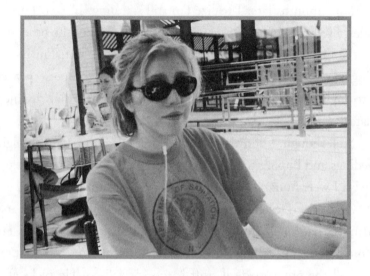

What Others Wrote
About My Transplant

No man is an island, entire of itself; every man is a piece
of the continent, a part of the main.
If a clod be washed away by the sea, Europe is the less,
as well as if a promontory were, as well as if a manor of
thy friend's or of thine own were: any man's death
diminishes me, because I am involved in mankind, and
therefore never send to know for whom the bell tolls;
it tolls for thee.
—John Donne

MARY SINCLAIR ROTHENBERG,
MY MOTHER

Life took an even more dramatic turn when Laura decided to
go active on the transplant list at Children's Hospital in Boston. It
was February of 2001 and the ringing of the telephone had a new
meaning, especially at night—we had been told that most organs
for transplantation become available at night. Now when the

phone rang, I wondered if this was THE CALL. The piercing sirens of the fire engines or the screeching cry of a police car in Brookline reminded me that this misfortune, whatever it was, could be connected with Laura. Her lungs were going to be related to another person's misfortune.

Time began to drag. We had originally been told that within a few weeks of her decision Laura would probably get the transplant call because with her transferred time from the New York Presbyterian Hospital list, she arrived as number two on the New England list for her blood type. I began to assure myself that it would take place on the date of a full or a new moon. Each month I checked the calendar to see when they were. The length of the wait was increasing. Laura was getting sicker and there were still no lungs. She was exasperated: how could she hang on to an interest in living when she was losing more and more energy with each new infection of these diseased lungs?

I was commuting from Brookline, Massachusetts, to New York and New York to Brookline mostly via Amtrak. The nights became shorter. I had watched the shoreline landscape along the northeastern coastline change from white to gray brown to light green to dark green as winter moved toward spring and then summer. The year before, Laura had been bounding around the Providence campus—even when not so well, she walked at a pace that was fast for me. Now she could barely walk along the pleasant sidewalks of Brookline at a pace slow enough to avoid the chain of coughing that physical activity precipitated.

Between one pre-transplant admission to the hospital and the next, and the next, there were many, many celebrations in the forms of visits to Laura in her apartment in Brookline and the hospital from friends coming far and wide. We spent time fixing up her apartment so that it would be welcoming for the friends who came to visit her there. The couches were recovered to make the living room more cheerful. And we hung many posters and pictures on the walls. These were accompanied, as time went on, with increasing numbers of Laura-made colorful origami cranes, which were strung one on top of the other (three or four on a string) and hung from the ceiling. The path of the flight of the cranes moved from her bedroom into the passage and then into the living room toward the front door.

There were many variations on visits with Laura. Sometimes there were both parents and Laura and friends. Or sometimes it was Laura and one parent and a friend. Or it was Laura and a friend or Laura and several friends. These visits were often cause for celebratory meals in the form of trying out all the local restaurants. We tried out the supermarkets, too. We developed some favorite hangouts in Brookline and Cambridge. We celebrated Easter in Brookline. We watched the Boston Marathon from the street in Brookline. And Laura enrolled in a watercolor class and helped out in an after-school program at the Park School in Boston. She created a transplant lottery. Friends each chose a date when they thought the transplant would really take place. Each one's choice was carefully written down on a calendar that was on the wall next to her bed below a collage of many meaningful pictures and mementos.

Our celebration of Laura's life has been going on for a long time and she has always been part of a larger family than just our nuclear family. This has not at all times been easy to accept. It started when she was very young. At ten weeks old, after Laura had finally recovered from her meconium ileus surgery, I went to pick her up from the hospital to bring her home for the first time. With me I had the clothes I had carefully selected for the exit from the hospital of my only child. But the nurses in the neonatal unit had all pitched in and purchased her an outfit with matching hat. There was no way for me to insist upon the clothes I had brought.

While we waited for the transplant I often felt the same. Each person was trying his or her best to help Laura get through the wait and each one was and is an important part of her life. Each was giving, and each one, no matter how they contacted Laura or how great or small their contribution, loved her and admired her courage and tried to help her, and each one had made a difference. And each time I realized this, I felt that we are all related and that it is really only in special circumstances like all the difficulties that Laura has faced and is still facing that we human beings begin to accept our relatedness.

DR. JON ROTHENBERG, MY FATHER

As a doctor I was long puzzled by the intensity of the emotional response in some patients to even minor symptoms or illnesses. That they were simply emotional didn't seem to explain this. Where did this intensity come from? At one point I had the thought that at such moments people touch the fear of death. It was like watching as my daughter first encountered the ocean as a mobile person, running along the edge of the tiny last waves with great excitement, over and over, why wouldn't she go in? And then realizing that perhaps she was feeling the whole ocean.

Beneath our conviction, our image, is there some vast terror? Could that be faced, transformed? By what? Or are there simply different forces, struggle, the need for balance?

These are the questions of someone who has lost something.

Why have I lost something? It seems to have to do with the intensity of the emotions surrounding the transplant, war, journey—it's all of those—and with the continuing uncertainty about what will happen next.

Of course the basis of this is that I care. I don't care so whole-heartedly simply because I am Laura's father. It's just worked out this way. Some think it is pathological—overconcern, depression, preoccupation, escape—but I don't. For the moment, this is what matters, whatever the consequences.

I knew something about intensity of emotions. I once thought that Keats was flowery: "O lift me as a wave, a leaf, a cloud. I fall upon the thorns of life. I bleed." Come on. But then I experienced romantic love, and saw these lines more as under-statements, and coarse—they couldn't match the flow. I have felt the joy of seeing the oneness of all things. Once, through inten-sity of emotion, I talked with a dying and out-of-touch friend over a distance. And I had a profound moment of understanding intensity, division, struggle, the brink of madness, and help . . . many years ago.

But during this year I have seen something else. Emotions so intense are unstable. I'm unable to control them. They burst out all over the place, narrowly, subjectively, vehemently, according to unconscious patterns from childhood kept more in check for years. One feature of this was particularly disturbing. My reaction to someone and that person's behavior was very strong. I expressed it unexpectedly at one point. It came to a kind of fixed attitude toward that person that I can only call hard-heartedness, something I had never experienced before. I refused my daughter's plea to make amends, with all she was going through, because to make amends would be betraying something. My own Middle East.

I've long known that, as a given, in my usual state, I have no faith. Or to put it another way, at moments when everything is stripped away, there is nothing to rely on. Much of the rest of the time, I am simply functioning automatically, being entirely passive or responding to demands. And there are also moments when I feel more as though I am free to be myself, however I am, because I am aware of something, some sense of existence, which is at that moment, without thinking about it, a basis of life. I have spent years trying to understand this better.

So, what has happened? Something in the emotions. I have fallen apart. I can no longer give the same answers I would have about the basis of meaning in my life. Nor do I know from where to come in daily events I am living. I feel something afoot, something that needs to be understood.

When I began to write, I thought I would be able to say

more. Perhaps later. Not that this questioning should in any way make less important what I have been privileged to witness surrounding Laura and the transplant, amid the panorama of so many emotions, of real caring, giving, friendship, humanity, and love.

Transplant Day, July 15, 2001. The beginning.

It seems hard to write with feeling about a moment so fully lived.

Either my wife or I or both had been in Boston for about five months. Sometimes Laura took the weekend alone and one of us went to join the other in New York. Sometimes the other came to Boston for the weekend before we switched. We had spent a week away in early July, the only time in the five months, to run a conference as we had done in early July for twenty years. But this time we had been sent home for the weekend. The friend who had been staying with Laura for a few weeks had left for a visit to Washington, and Laura's three college roommates of the last year had chosen to get together at her apartment.

Laura was getting sicker. She'd had a fungal infection of her port requiring surgical removal and lengthy intravenous treatment. And she'd had an episode of intractable hemoptysis, bleeding from the lungs that didn't stop, halted luckily by an intravenous embolization procedure. The hospitalizations for antibiotics for her chronic lung infection were not making the difference they should have. And she was sicker than anyone realized. It wasn't until the surprise from the pathology report on the old lungs that we realized how sick she had been.

And the transplant wasn't coming. The team was supposed to do up to four or five lung transplants a year, but we'd been months at the top of their list and several months at the top of the New England list for Laura's blood type. The lung transplant medical director spoke of an "organ drought."

We had expected a wait of two to three months. Laura had withdrawn from the winter semester at school in part because she thought she would not have time to complete any courses. When she wasn't in the hospital, Laura did some student teaching, tried an art class, and watched favorite television programs. She couldn't read much. Many friends visited. We went to restaurants. But it was getting thin. The three months' recovery time we wanted so she would be ready to return to Brown in the fall wasn't going to happen. The medical team didn't understand why that mattered in the scale of things. But Laura was taking the transplant not to survive, but to be able to live her life, a life inextricably bound up with people. She had boldly taken a third-floor walk-up off-campus apartment for the fall at a time when she could hardly walk up one flight. And there was only a certain time period for her to remain in contact with her friends at school, who would be moving on. Transplant is not a time to make new friends. And then there was us. Laura would have been in college, seeing little of us. She was ready and anxious to lead her own life. It was hard, particularly for me, and for me as a doctor to be enough in the background.

But how to convey what this really meant to me. I recall the first minute, February 6, 1981, standing in the parent area of the New York Hospital Neonatal Intensive Care Unit where a very long hall stretched along the length of the unit from the entrance, standing with my wife and her parents, watching the doctor, my classmate, take this long walk slowly—one of the most difficult things he's had to do he said later, because there were two likely causes of the abdominal obstruction relieved by her emergency surgery on the third day of her life, one with consequences lasting three months, which he had thought it would be and pictured himself giving us the good news, and the other cystic fibrosis. And then he told us, my knees bending almost to the floor before I made myself stand up, being the only one who knew what it meant. It had hit me all at once, some impression of the difficulty of her whole life.

The phone rang at 5 A.M. Laura was surrounded by her roommates, who were very excited. I was focused on getting there. The big thing was to see her before she went in.

The decision to accept the lungs is a complicated one. During our wait the transplant team had several times been offered lungs that they turned down (we always found out afterward). First there was the history: the age of the patient, cause of death, associated diseases, hospital course. The transplant surgeon, for example, preferred not to put the lungs of a sixty-five-year-old into a twenty-year-old patient. If the history was promising, the surgical harvest team, under Dr. Shamburger, would go to the donor hospital, by jet plane if necessary, to look at the patient's chart and chest X ray, and then perform a bronchoscopy to look at the interior of the lungs. With these results, the lead transplant surgeon, Dr. Lillehei, would decide.

Then, who to offer the lungs to? Laura was among the O blood type of people who could only receive lungs from O blood type donors, but those lungs could also go to people with blood types

A, B, and AB, who had separate lists. This was the one part of the process we hadn't queried. Someone later told us—a rumor—that the lungs had been offered first to someone else, who wasn't available, presumably from one of the other three lists, but this hardly mattered. Then, time-wise, there would be the question of which organ team gets to harvest first, etc., as several organs are likely to have been donated. Even after the lungs are harvested and brought back to Laura's hospital, there would be the final inspection before going ahead. We didn't know exactly where in the process Laura had been called, although we knew that the lungs are never harvested until the recipient is at the hospital and medically cleared to receive them.

It wasn't difficult. I had been planning on going to Boston and was almost completely packed. I had been carrying back and forth a heavy second suitcase containing what papers and equipment would be needed for an extensive stay, which I had not unpacked for the weekend.

But it was Sunday. The first shuttle from New York to Boston was on US Air; on Sunday it didn't leave till nine o'clock. We still might have time. I made the reservation and we took a taxi to the airport. But there was a problem. The US Air shuttle was changing its security vendor, this being the last day for the old vendor, and no one had showed up. There was no one to screen the carry-on luggage. So after a cell phone call secured a reservation on the 9:30 Delta shuttle, we cabbed over and made the flight. But we were less sure about arriving in time.

Laura would not be alone. One great friend of Laura's, who lived closer than we did, drove at 90 miles an hour and would be the first to arrive to join the roommates. Another woman, a family friend, who had provided the apartment we had been using in Boston, took a private plane from Fisher's Island, and arrived next. There were friends in Boston and Brown students who were in Providence for the summer, an hour away.

One high school classmate who had been determined to come was in Woodstock for the weekend at the home of another high school classmate, who upon hearing the news promptly woke up her father and asked him to drive the five hours to Boston immediately, which he did. He missed seeing Laura by about fifteen minutes, gave his well wishes, then drove back to his wife. The friend who had gone away for the weekend had come to stay with Laura so she could be there for the transplant; no one had her number, and she had inadvertently left her cell phone off. When she arrived later in the day, she was still upset.

Of course, the beginning really didn't matter; it was going to be a long haul, first weeks, and then, as it turned out, months.

We were lucky it was Sunday. The surgical Family Waiting Area at Children's Hospital in Boston is two large rooms. On weekdays, as we were later to know all too well, these are almost filled with parents and a few friends. Where would there have been room for Mary and Jon and Debra and Ann and Lauren and Courtney and Kat and Jess and Emma and Lucy and Rebecca and Tiffany and Vicki and EB and Louella and Hentyle and Ben and Ryan and Ali and Brooke and Adam? And Kate, four years post–lung transplant, also for CF. Playing cards, working at the computer, sleeping. Pictures and more pictures. Laura wanted pictures of everything. Debra persuaded the transplant coordinator to take pictures of the old and new lungs in the operating room with Ann's digital camera. So everyone was able to look at the pictures on the digital monitor while Laura was in the OR. This hadn't been done before, and we later supplied requested enlargements to the leader of the harvest team and the transplant surgeon.

When the surgical team finally met with the four most senior in waiting, they stressed the need to limit visitors to Laura in the first week of immunosuppression. It turned out that none of those waiting except us four would be able to see her. So we had a big meeting, everyone together, and I talked, and Mary talked, and Kate, the one who'd had a transplant, talked. And seven or eight of Laura's friends divided Laura's list and used all the cell phones to spread the news. It was of course impossible to convey what it had been like to meet with the transplant team, what it was like to be in the small room with them, after the long surgery, the state they were in—words like exhilaration or excitement or pride or fulfillment fall way short.

When the plane landed, we didn't call. It seemed to matter a great deal that we see her. We didn't know if we'd see her again, or see her again as herself. Mary went straight to the hospital while I gathered the luggage before taking a second taxi. I knew the hospital all too well, and where to go.

I had my luggage on the special fold-up two-wheeler I'd been using for train travel between New York and Boston these months, and it was quite heavy and bulky. Seeing unexpectedly so many people in the waiting room of the ICU, where Laura was kept pre-transplant, I headed without saying anything toward an open

closet where I could stow my luggage out of everyone's way. Our
friend asked to take the cart, but I went ahead, thinking no one
else knew how to maneuver it. I was completely unprepared for
the force with which she then tried to take the cart from me, and
with which I resisted. Afterward, she said she'd known Laura was
about to be taken, and she wanted to be sure I saw her. This must
have been made more poignant by her own hesitation. After making such an effort to get there, seeing Laura with others, she had
felt shy to push herself forward, and actually didn't spend time
with Laura before the surgery.

Our friend led me toward Laura. She was surrounded—the
transplant coordinator, her friends. We had made it. She saw me.
I could see she was in a good state. She was ready. I was with her.
It was enough. Someone handed me Laura's cell phone. It was a
call from one of her great supporters, an anesthesiologist and former ICU head at Babies' Hospital in New York, who was to be on
the phone daily during Laura's post-transplant days—an important call because I didn't know what he knew. Just at that moment
I was taken aback by the sudden appearance of the chief transplant
surgeon, who wanted to let me know what was happening. I felt I
didn't give either of them enough attention. The lungs had looked
good at the bronchoscopy; they were about to harvest them, and
Laura would go to the surgical suite now.

And then I heard my name. I turned around, and there was
Laura, offering me, completely unexpected, the sweetest hug of
my whole life. She was in herself, relaxed, so alive, so open. I
stepped back. I watched the nurse come for her stretcher, and
followed it, and took pictures as she was wheeled across the

ICU to the entryway, surrounded by the throng of well-wishers in celebration as she went so gently in triumph to face the rest of her life.

EMILY TURNER,
HIGH SCHOOL FRIEND ──────────────

I received a phone message to call Rebecca from my room-mate and knew right away that it was "the call." But I tried to stay calm and quickly dialed Rebecca at home. No answer.

Called her cell phone. No answer. Okay, okay, stay calm. Call Laura's cell phone. If she did go in to get lungs, she most likely left some sort of special message on her machine. Rings once. Rings twice. Come on message, I just want to know for sure! "Hello"— wait this is not a message, this is a man's voice. "Hello," I respond. It's Dr. Rothenberg. A moment of silence, and then I ask, "Is Laura home?" Quick chuckle from her dad, and then he tells me you have gone to the hospital and he is just picking up a few last things for you. I am so excited; I am jumping up and down while I am on the phone. Your father and I are yelling to each other over the phone. (I think he may have been spastically jumping as well.) He has to go, and I am left to wait.

I run next door to tell my friend Farrar. I scream so loudly that her roommates think there is someone beating me. We jump up and down, I cry, we hug. It was great. Then I go home, jump in my car and drive to Kiki's. Kiki is also from New York and was very close to Sophie Laumont who passed away in high school from CF. Again I go through the screaming, jumping, crying thing. By now I have had an hour to think about what is happening to Laura in Boston and I begin to get scared. I cannot stop moving.

Even now, as I type this, I have a sense of overwhelming urgency that can only be manifested through uncontrollable movement. My blood was pumping, my endorphins flowing and my emotions on overload. I went home. I tried to do schoolwork, but could not function. One of my guy friends offered to take me to the driving range, but I refused to leave my phone. So I paced. I drove my five roommates crazy. There was nothing they could do to get me out of my mania—one minute rejoicing, the next silenced with fear. I thought about driving to Boston. I called Hayley, Rebecca, and Tiffany obsessively. And when I could not reach them, I called Rebecca's mom. I called her so many times she told me, "If there is any news from Becky, I will call you. But we need to keep the line open."

By the end of the afternoon I was exhausted, but could not sleep. I had sweated so much during the day that I had to shower twice. I considered having a drink but decided not to. I continued to wait. I watched *Duets* with Gwyneth Paltrow one and a half times. I smoked three packs of cigarettes, I vomited.

At 5 P.M., I realized it was my sister's twenty-second birthday so I gave her a quick call. I missed her but left a message. I believe it was, "Oh my God, Laura got the best birthday present ever. Love ya. Em." Not so much sense. Finally I received word from Rebecca, and later her mother that Laura was in recovery and the surgery had gone well. I was relieved. (At this point I could not begin to think about the actual recovery. Laura had new lungs and that was enough for me for one day.) I had a few more smokes and then went for drinks with my roommates. According to them, I was "more of a jackass than other nights."

DR. ADAM VELLA, CURRENTLY AN ER FELLOW AT LOS ANGELES CHILDREN'S HOSPITAL

Laura's going to get a transplant. First reaction: fear. Of course, I pretty much only see the ones that don't do well, but that's why I'm afraid. Normally I'm able to put a little distance between myself and the unfortunate child suffering, but Laura's more than my patient, she's my friend. In fact, long ago we stopped acting as doctor/patient and started down the path of buddies. The drop-ins during her admits: "Laura, why's your room not set up yet?" or "Dude, you gotta stop playing the *Les Mis!*" or "I'm so sorry you have that intern, he needs a little work, I'll talk to him . . ." or "Damn, you're on a major solumedrol swing; I'll stop by when you're feeling better."

So when most people take a little break in college to do some traveling or just hang out, Laura takes a break to have someone else's lungs placed inside her chest. Starts with elation, the waiting has ended. Then onto the roller coaster. There's so much going on that I'm pretty much unable to keep up with the developments. I get the e-mails, try to absorb the crucial stuff, and give a call when things aren't going well. Uh-oh, PFTs dropping, I've seen it before, and so soon after transplant, I don't want to think about where this is going. . . . Rejection/infection/rejection/infection somebody just make a call already! Don't really understand how she functions at all.

I see her for coffee in NYC; she's breathing fast, definitely retracting, looks very similar to my pre-transplant friend Laura Rothenberg! What's the point of getting a new set of lungs if they're not going to help you oxygenate and ventilate? This is bullshit! I don't want to get caught clinically assessing her, but she knows I'm looking. Sick children always know the deal, they see the looks in our eyes, and immediately intuit their situation somehow, don't really understand it myself. Laura is not a child, though. She is an intelligent young poet/writer who fully understands the precariousness of her situation. That for me is the worst part. She knows more than myself about her chances, the numbers. She has said good-bye to more friends with CF in her short lifetime. Just a few weeks ago she lost another good friend from Babies'. On she goes, fighting.

DEBRA, MY GODMOTHER

I generally try to keep somewhat of a running memoir of events, and the ways in which I take them in, but, ironically, some of the most potent ones do not allow me the time in which to do so. I would say that the events of July 2001 would fall under this category. And so once again I thank you for the opportunity to collect some reflections and put them down on paper.

One always thinks of the preparation time when a big event is to occur. We carry the necessary information with us, and slowly, throughout our day, we fool ourselves into thinking we are getting ready. Perhaps it is not a total misconception, for how do we know how we would be without this time?

The call came at five in the morning and there was an element of surprise due to the hour, but it took only a minute to hoist myself out of bed and get dressed, get in the car, and proceed to set the land speed record for a woman from New York to Boston.

I can only say that I knew all along it would be all-consuming, but perhaps not in the way that I imagined. There was the time spent with you before you went in, and that was mostly taken up with the business of the team that was prepping you and just being a presence for whatever was needed.

Seeing you actually going in was a bit of a high, since you were so ready and willing; almost a relief. The fear sets in later, when there is time to do that most unproductive of practices, think.

Your parents were of first concern. Did they have what they needed and the support they would need in the time to come? Your friends, arriving in hordes, were the next concern, and your father seemed to have a handle on how to deal with them. I suppose that after years of watching you and how you made your way through the world, all of us have at least an idea of how you like to have things run.

When the surgery was over and you were moving into what seemed at the time to be the hardest part of the program, there appeared to be a plan that consisted of concentric circles of care and support. I think somewhere along the line, the combination of sleeplessness and stress took its toll and we all suffered a bit from the confusion that can come with it.

I know that I never lost track of why I was there. It has never been a defined relationship, you and I; we seem to move freely between different roles and it has always worked that way just fine. I knew all along that I have been there not only for you, but also for myself and for your grandfather—the connection that brought us together to begin with. In the roughest times, I try to keep him in front of me to remember the joy with which he beheld you.

You struggled mightily in those first few days, and it was a constant decision as to how to stay out of the way and help at the same time. Some moments were more successful than others were. You would wake, or half wake and want as much information as you could get and then something else would take hold and you would be off working that out in a world that only you can know.

My feeling was that you were in a world where there were fires to be put out, battles to be fought, and very little time to worry about the trivialities that can fill one's days. Day in and day out, you were working. Your frustrations and triumphs were clear. My place in the events of each day could change very rapidly, and often I didn't pay enough attention and would get caught up short. But I know this: I observed you, your parents, and those whom you love and who love you working together in all the ways they knew to get you on your feet and ready for a new phase of life. A team is a team because of their spirit, not always because they play perfectly together all the time.

So there I am, a player on Team Laura, and on my own, well, I carry you in my heart each and every day. I can say that with 100 percent honesty. I think of you and place myself with you each and every day. I don't know if there will be a time when that changes, but I guess in a way I hope so. I know that it is still a struggle. A complex, and sometimes baffling combination of desire, urgency, and the need to relax into some sort of "normalcy." I do not often look back—in fact, as a rule, ever—so forgive my lack of detail. It seems that I am still in the same head that I have always been with you and will continue to be.

JESSICA WATERS, COLLEGE FRIEND

My dad once told me that the road of life is full of little bumps, and that some bumps are bigger than others, but that he was sure I could overcome this one. I don't remember which bump he was talking about at the time, but I do remember what he said. It's funny how something corny like that can be so true; but then, I suppose that in order to be repeated enough times to become trite, an expression must hold some truth. "Big bump" you call your bowel obstruction and subsequent operation. It makes me think of my life; I have yet to spend a night inside a hospital. I can't even begin to imagine what it is like for you. Can you imagine what it is like for me?

I met this girl in my Hard Choices section; she obviously had a bad case of bronchitis or something. Pretty and self-assured, she presented her ideas clearly and confidently. In contrast to myself, she seemed to know what she was talking about, but unlike with some of the other students, her knowledge didn't make me feel inferior. I would later learn why she seemed to understand medicine like no one else in that small room.

Fun. Spirited. Spoiled. A real New Yorker. Obnoxious. Wise. Social butterfly. A great friend. Always the center of attention. Poised. Articulate. Open. Mature. Amazing. These are the words I used to describe my new friend. I remember the night that we sat in her dorm room and discussed random facts about our pasts—how could you know someone without knowing where they came from? I was so excited when she asked me to live with her. I was flattered that someone so special would pick me.

Though I watched her body fight its losing battle against the disease, it was the psychological (spiritual?) struggle that captured me and through which she earned my admiration, my respect. Sometimes it seemed as though she would go under, and, not knowing what to say or do, I despaired with her. But I couldn't get over the fact that she never did cave in; somehow, she was winning.

This summer, she waited, a triumph in itself. I watched her being rolled toward the operating room, her eyes glazed from the drugs but her smile bright and excited. As I lay on the chairs in the OR waiting room, I thought of the doctors next door and wished that I could do as much for her as they could. I thought of her chest, open and exposed to the outside world, and of how the tiniest mishap could break that fragile body. If there was a God, this was his moment, I thought to myself.

I would like to say that now, with the surgery successfully completed and school in sight, it's over, but it continues. Every prayer of thanks to the God who may or may not exist (whether he does or not, I'm definitely covering all my bases) for the miracle that occurred in that operating room is followed by a fervent request for more. Give her more experiences, more smiles, more birthday parties, more classes at Brown. And give me more experience, more smiles, birthday parties, and classes with her. I feel lucky to know someone like her. I hope she feels lucky to know me.

LUCY BOYLE,
HIGH SCHOOL FRIEND ———————————————

before

like a baby you took
my fingers in your fist,
holding tight, testing your
strength. your body curled
on the gurney, you were calm,
so calm and so wise, a knowing
cat. the smile like a string
of beads. maybe it was your meds, but
in that moment it felt like you
were holding me up.

during

i walk through air-stained tunnels
of hospital halls as surgeons
navigate your bones your arteries
past your aorta down to your
dying lungs

the fifth-floor connector has wombful
pink walls and windows so big
they let in spheres of light
while walking through I stop

to look out through the glass
and rain shakes like powder
through a July sun sky

during

wanting to be useful
the digital pictures of the new
lungs, the old lungs

how can i sit still

during

i walk on a raked stage:
the fact of its descent down,
the grainy paint designed to stop
our falls, nothing can
compete with you in the OR
your body cut open, your ribs
yawning like a red mouth to receive
lungs from a body just stopped

after

we didn't realize that the fight didn't end
here, that for a week you would swim

without water every hour and then
return to some subterranean sphere

through the ICU glass you seem
to melt from wax as the days pass
each time I visit I am allowed
a look

after

you know how much and
how little it can mean to
write a poem like this one—
lines broken and re-broken,
short but trying to cover
the distance from the right
lung to the left eye

DR. STEVEN STYLIANOS, MY SURGEON IN NEW YORK (DIRECTOR, REGIONAL PEDIATRIC TRAUMA PROGRAM, CHILDREN'S HOSPITAL OF NEW YORK-PRESBYTERIAN)

The most palpable emotion I recall is wondering how children and adolescents with CF can cope with the news that their friends die one by one with the same disease they are battling. How can you not wonder when it will be your turn to be eulogized?

When Laura was listed for transplant, I hoped that she would be spared the regret of waiting too long prior to getting listed, as had many of her friends with CF. Laura's transplant and recovery were a celebration of courage and wisdom in a young lady who has had a profound effect on me as a pediatric surgeon and as a friend.

GENEVIEVE LOWRY, CHILD LIFE SPECIALIST AT COLUMBIA

How did your transplant affect me? I am not so sure I can truly say. I try not to spend that much time thinking about it. When one works with children who may die, one sometimes puts that out of one's mind. It makes it impossible to be yourself and inhibits personal connections with the individual children.

The problem between you and me is that we've crossed too

many lines. I pride myself on my ability to maintain boundaries, because without them I am unable successfully to do the work I love. However, I must protect myself. I tell myself these are not my children, and yet in order to gain each child's trust, I must give of myself personally.

This is how it all began. I don't even remember the first time we met. It seems as if I always just knew you. I always thought it was when Gina died that our relationship changed, but thinking about it now we were always close from the beginning.

So, where do I file Laura in my professional life? You are too young to be a friend, it would be too hard to think of you as a sister, but you're not just an ordinary patient, either. So during that time you were in Boston it was like floundering. If I had a definition for us, I would have known what to do, where my place was. I was so grateful for the calls from your parents. They made me feel a part of it all. You never know, sometimes when people leave the hospital they want nothing to do with you, to forget it all. Or when in crisis, I may not be the one they think to call. I try so hard to keep my own "work" relationships in perspective, it is just another way of protecting myself. Never think you're too important to a family. I never knew if I should call or if you would be mad when you found out that I didn't.

The hardest time for me personally wasn't so much the transplant but the PTLD, the complications of transplant. I remember thinking about the rippling effect your death would have had on the medical center. The numbers of people who would have been affected. That was when I lost it. Thank God that didn't

happen. It is hard for me to imagine, though. I continue to picture you in this world. If I hold on to those images they become
real. Deep down I knew you would be okay, and I still believe
that. I used to think of Javier as the sole survivor, but now I know
it's you.

BRYAN L. DOERRIES,
BOYFRIEND ————————————————————

The Problem with Symmetry

Then, she pulled back her shirt
   and showed me the
scars, pink and raised,
   a landscape of abandoned
railroads, cross ties, buttons,
   the lashes of an invisible whip.

To know is to suffer knowledge,
   to learn the lesson twice,
thrice, and then forget, only
   to learn again through suffering.

Before the procedure, she began to shake,
   like an ancient prophet, blessed
with the falling sickness, but after
   she rattled like a subway car
barreling over the Brooklyn bridge
   toward the land of shadows, over
the river of forgetfulness, terminating
   on a sacred island at the end
of the line, only to return between
   breath and the breathing.

The problem with symmetry lies
   in the mendacity of wholeness:

the gaze of Narcissus, the blinding
    of synecdoche, where a part becomes
whole, but never wholly part of the image
    she sees when she looks in the mirror:

cascading cicatrices the color
    of bruised turnips, jutting
numbness, hieroglyphic histories
      inscribed with a knife,
fragmented, detached, beautiful.

The problem with symmetry is that
    it doesn't *really* exist. In the same
way the earth isn't *really* round,
      but rotates all the same. The human form,
Mr. DaVinci, is the last place to look
    for an equiangular spiral.

EB KELLY, FRIEND SINCE FIFTH GRADE

I must admit that even though I knew how dangerous and scary the surgery was, sitting in the waiting room on July 15, 2001, I felt hugely impatient for it to be done and for her to come out. I mean, everything with Laura feels like it has been a battle against the impossible, the improbable, the unlikely, so I treated her lung transplant in much the same way. Yes, it was a huge deal. Yes, it could not turn out okay. But by that point, the fact that she had waited around all that time for the lungs seemed the real challenge, and now came the easy part of being given them. I remembered the tough time that my cousin Kate had just after her surgery, but that quickly faded to the background when I thought about how vibrant and active she is now. Laura just needed to get the lungs, hang out in the ICU for a bit, and then she would be on her feet, like never before.

I felt no nostalgia for those dumb old lungs. (In fact, my most vivid memory of the waiting process was saying good-bye to Laura in June after I had been in Boston visiting for a weekend. As I hugged her good-bye, she suggested I squeeze extra hard in case it was the last time I hugged those lungs. I remember so vividly how little her ribs felt against my arms, and how I had no remorse at all if that was the last I would get to hold those diseased old lungs.)

Anyway, back to transplant time. So as I said, once I had gotten over the initial shock, the day of the surgery and the day after seemed to me just one more part of the waiting process. Wait until she's out and then back and better than ever. I went back to New York, proudly told everyone I met about my friend and her new lungs, and then got set to come back the next weekend to see her when she was conscious.

I flew back up to Boston the following weekend, for two days filled with more hanging out in the ICU, punctuated most excitingly by a lengthy bath of the patient involving an enema bag, a bed pan, and one of Laura's roommates from Brown. Amazing the things we do for love. I was so happy to see and talk to Laura, and though she was still all wired up I felt like the new her was about to take the scene.

Yet only after returning home that Sunday night did I really let my emotions catch up with me. I flew home and headed out

to some cheesy movie with my family that night. We decided to
walk to the theater, and headed down Lexington. When we got to
66th Street, all of a sudden tears welled up in my eyes. For it was
at that moment, looking at Laura's house, that I finally realized
just how close I had been to losing such an important part of my
life, and how much Laura truly means to me. As we passed Laura's
home, I just thought of all the memories that we shared in that
place. New York was not the same without her there, and it would
always be like that for me. For the first time (I think ever) in my
friendship with Laura, I realized just how unable I would be to go
on without her. Yes, theoretically, there has always been the possibility of losing her. But never had it been as palpable to me as
when I saw the literal reminders of all that we had shared together.

And at that moment I became more scared than I had ever
been at any time in Laura's sickness. The physical manifestation
of Laura's home, juxtaposed against the ever-looming possibility
that I might never see her again made me feel vulnerable and
afraid. I could not stand not having her in my life. That was completely unacceptable. I suppose it was at that moment I realized
what it means to love someone so deeply that they become a part
of you. And that is what I remember about Laura's transplant.
The discovery that a part of Laura had been permanently transplanted into me—a part so vital I could not exist without it.

AUNT JUDY

I never knew my oldest brother very well when we were growing up because he was ten years older than I.

Jon and Mary had lived together for some years. I remember the day he proposed as if it were yesterday. When the family called, I yelled and screamed on the phone that they should stop teasing me because I didn't believe it. Finally, my other brother had to get on the phone to tell me it was really true. The wedding was a lovely celebration on a windy and drizzly day in Riverdale, New York.

Laura was born on February 3, 1981. But the answer to the question about how mother and baby were doing changed after a couple days. Laura developed an intestinal blockage and had surgery at four days. Diagnosis, cystic fibrosis. I didn't really comprehend what that would mean, but I knew it wasn't good. How hard for Jon and Mary. Laura was a fighter from the start. Otherwise, she would have gone the route of the other fetuses. But this one—she wanted to survive. She wanted a life. I knew that when she was in her first week of life.

I cannot remember when I first met her, but I think she was toddling around by then. I lived halfway across the country, had just started working, and had few resources. But I was sent a picture that was taken when she was sitting, probably when she was eight months old. Her hands were held in a praying position and she looked out and upward with her almost-larger-than-life eyes. An old soul. One with some kind of destiny.

Jon, Mary, and Laura traveled to visit my parents around the Christmas holiday every year. When she was four years old, I happened to intersect with them in Florida for a couple days. The morning they were leaving, Laura played with me on the floor of the middle bedroom. There wasn't much space and there weren't many toys still unpacked. She acted out a sick child going to the hospital by ambulance. She didn't know much about her illness. I don't even think she knew the name of it. Just that she had to take a huge pill before she ate. The play was otherworldly and uncanny. I knew she was preparing herself.

Jump forward to the first time I spent a beach vacation with Jon and Mary before I married. Laura was coughing, in a way I had never heard her cough before. Somehow I knew she wasn't going to stop coughing. Her illness had been a bit on the back burner for as long as possible. I knew that those days were numbered.

I don't remember when she went on the transplant list. I just remember that my mother told me about it. The idea was to put her name on the list in case she ever needed a transplant.

She flourished academically. She wrote unbelievably beautiful poetry that revealed the deepness of her thought about her illness. No longer the naive toddler. Now sicker. More frequent hospitalizations. I read every newspaper article about CF patients surviving against all odds for a long time with hope. Perhaps to help myself have hope.

Jon called and asked me to come to Laura's high school graduation. I never attended any other nieces' or nephews' high school graduations. Jon explained that they wanted to make this special for Laura because perhaps it might be her last graduation. I immediately agreed to come and devoted my visit to making her celebration memorable. Laura had arranged a special party at a restaurant with hospital and other supporters. I prepared a speech about her strengths and spoke for the family. I also made her a couple family tree posters. I started the speaking after dinner. Jon and Mary were worried that no one would speak so I had been pegged to get the ball rolling. It worked. One after one, nurses, doctors, residents, and interns spoke about all they had learned from my little one. I was so proud.

She went to Brown and made it through a year and a half. She decided to take a leave of absence and go active on the transplant list. I was afraid, afraid we would lose her. The longer the wait, the scarier it became. Long before, Laura asked me to come see her after she had the transplant. I was afraid I would never have the chance. I wondered if I should go see her anyway. I thought that perhaps her life was slowly ebbing away. I wanted to see her before she died.

Finally, Jon called with the news that she was going into surgery—they had new lungs for her. He explained the procedure, the odds, and how everything was set up at the hospital. I desperately wanted to do something to help, but I was all the way across the country. Part of me felt jealous of the two friends who were helping Jon and Mary at the hospital and part of me felt so thankful that they were there. I called every day to see how things were going. One call was answered by one of the friends. She talked about how much Jon was stressing out. I suddenly knew how I could help.

Over the years, I had come to spend more time with Jon than any of my other siblings. He was fun. And my relationship with Laura was not going to last for my entire lifetime. Now he needed support. Badly. So I changed the nature of my calls. I called to ask him how he was doing. He was surprised when I asked him the first time. I explained that I wanted to be there for him because I was his sister and I knew this had to be hard on him. He talked a little.

When I did go visit about six weeks post-transplant, he picked me up at the airport and we stayed at a motel before crossing over to Fisher's Island the next day. He spent almost two hours talking, explaining, and venting about the difficulties he and Laura were experiencing. I don't think his feelings dissipated, but I knew he was calmer the next morning. I had found a way to help. In so doing, I had finally bridged a gap I had felt my whole life. I felt emotionally connected with Jon in a way I never had before. I never anticipated that Laura's transplant would provide the opportunity for this to occur. But it did and I am grateful. He can still be a pain in the butt, but I have seen his vulnerabilities in a way I never experienced in the past.

I had the experience of pure joy watching Laura ride a bicycle for the first time in years at Fisher's Island. We had a chance to talk about her experience of the pre-transplant and post-transplant phases of her life when I drove her to Boston for a doctor's appointment. We spoke about her awareness that she had been fading—it wasn't the easiest subject to discuss, but I felt ever so relieved to speak about it openly.

Things were going swimmingly up until that point. Then, complication after complication after complication. Each time I heard about the newest physical mess, I tried hard to remember the angel with the almost-larger-than-life eyes who had so much hope, who had a mission to accomplish, and I tried to believe that somehow her body would see its way through this. At several points, I imagined myself at her funeral. Standing in front of a packed church and, again, speaking for my family. Reading my favorite Laura Rothenberg poem, the one about her party. I do want to do that, but the image was wrong. It isn't time yet.

One day, Laura called and talked to me about a psychic reading she had over the telephone. It gave her hope and it confirmed what I had sensed—it isn't her time now. The physical struggles are going to be hard. That won't really change. But she is going to be with us for a longer period of time. I am sure of it. This is Laura, the fighter since the day she was conceived, the fighter who hasn't finished her mission yet. It is hard to trust what I sense, but the transplant has given Laura more time. It is hard to watch her struggle, but, as she has always known, the fight is worth it. I remain in awe of her ability to fight and love her the more for the frailty and vulnerability she has shown in this last year. I have learned much about the human spirit from having been through this experience with her.

BEN TORPEY, COLLEGE FRIEND

I look her straight in the chest, trying, I suppose, to catch a glimpse of the action: patched tissue, twisted vessels and veins and fleshy white stuff and whatever else has been ripped apart, sewn back together, the scars, the hysterical white blood cells (Get these things out of here! What the hell *are* these things?), the immunosuppressants trying to keep everyone calm (Nothing to see here folks, keep it movin'). Drugs swirling, telling each other and everything else what to do and when; it must be chaos, and I want to see.

Shrink me and give me one of those little pods you can ride through the bloodstream in, the ones that corner like a dream on the giant network of red rivers. Set my bearings for New Lungs

One and Two, full throttle warp speed, then cut me loose and let me look around. Maybe then I will understand what all this means because "I just had a Double Lung Transplant" and all the medical jargon she's spewing doesn't explain the fact that Laura is looking like Laura, getting sauce on her face like Laura, breathing like Laura, with lungs that are not hers, or are becoming hers, or are just lungs, not belonging to her or anyone, but breathing nonetheless.

It's early August and I'm leaving the country for most of a year in a few weeks. We meet in the air-conditioned lobby of her apartment building. She is thinner, with chopped hair and a big smile. She looks good. I don't think I was expecting her to look this good. Also, she is breathing. In, and it's so good to see you, and out and in. This is how she breathes. It won't be easy, she is saying. The first year is the hardest. We eat pasta in a sunny café in Brookline. I sit across from my friend and watch her chest. In and out and chew and in and slurp and swallow and out. All at once, without thinking. That is how we breathe.

DR. DAVID OLSEN, THIRD-YEAR RESIDENT, BOSTON CHILDREN'S HOSPITAL

I thought that I would take a slightly different approach to the question of "what's it been like to be involved with Laura and her transplant." The "and" is important there because clearly there is more to Laura than the transplant. It has been a little odd to be a rather minor player in Laura's health pre- and post-transplant.

Not being a pulmonologist, but being Laura's resident (emphasis on the possessive), our first encounter was really about my learning the nuts and bolts of CF care from a seasoned veteran. I quickly realized, though, that I was probably doing more good as a friend, in addition to being a caregiver.

The richness of my interaction with Laura has come not from the medicine but from getting to know her over the bumpy path of the last twelve months (or so). The ins and outs and ups and downs, successes and setbacks of CF/lung transplant don't register for me in terms of lab values, CT scan results, or pulmonary function tests. We seem to use those things to set the table for our interactions, sort of an ice-breaker at a familiar dinner party. But once those things are stated, we are left with the substance of what is human and relational. What quickly takes on importance is not the day's PFTs, yesterday's CT scan, or even the wonders of enumerating Laura's medical history.

The real gold comes from looking at the latest knitting creations, planning to send a skunk pill to a little friend, talking about classes at Brown, sharing lunch (which used to be the all-nutritious fudgsicle), or hearing about "special friends." I realize that I kind of like not being Laura's resident, but rather one of the many people she would I hope refer to as a friend. Years from now, I am sure that I will forget the nuances of CF care and its hospital management. However, I will never forget the simply fabulous hairdos, paper cranes, fudgsicle lunches, and the look of excitement in the eyes of a college sophomore having to select classes and ponder her return to Providence.

If anything, CF has been the means to an end for me—it's

been a free pass into the sanctum of somebody else's life. And aside from the ups and downs, disappointments, setbacks and physical victories, the warmth of friendship that I feel walking into a now familiarly decorated hospital room is cherished.

MARIANN, NURSE ON THE TRANSPLANT FLOOR

I am writing about my impressions and observations as an RN in the experience of Laura R. and her lung transplant. I remember my initial meeting with Laura, vividly. I approached room 817, "A Room of Her Own" and proceeded to assess Laura's vital signs and respiratory status. Laura meanwhile was busy in her multitasking way. As she talked on the phone with her laptop computer open and on, she held out her arm for her b/p and her left pointer finger for the oxygen saturation clip. She never missed a word or thought in her phone conversation and her b/p and O2 saturation were excellent. I thought, "Oh, boy" a real busy, involved gal. I then took a few moments to enjoy the interior design of her room. A vintage shaded lamp, musical cell phone, multicolored origami cranes hanging from IV poles, inspirational posters and pictures, pictures, pictures of family and friends. So unique, so Laura!

Our relationship has continued over the past nine months as Laura has been admitted many times with complicated medical and surgical challenges to her post-transplant life. We have shared many up days and many down days. Through each of these experiences I have been impressed with Laura's courage, open communication style, sense of humor and intelligence. Her honesty and courage as her own advocate has grown and blossomed and I have felt privileged to be involved in her care. In closing I would like to share a verse that I associate with Laura R.

No coward soul is mine
No trembler in the world's storm-troubled sphere
I see Heaven's glories shine
And faith shines equal, arming me from fear.
—Emily Bronte, 1846

WILL SCHUTT, HIGH SCHOOL FRIEND

Most of it took place over the phone. It's been our custom since leaving for college. She calls and I call back; I call and she picks up; she calls and I'm not there; she calls and I'm there.

There's not too much "coming over" anymore, though I visited Laura once before the operation, while she waited in Boston for the page. The apartment was full of origami cranes she'd been making, as she'd told me; her room was made up the way it always is—in the hospital, at home, in Providence, now, I'm sure. There are always pictures of new and old friends. There are quotes, animals, and Eeyore. And yet I remember thinking that it wasn't the way I'd imagined it.

I guess because she told me over the phone, because of my naïveté (Laura often lists her assorted ailments, the drugs she takes for each, the possible operations, but I'm never able to keep them straight in my head), because I'm still stupidly a bit carefree, because, in my mind, Laura has always been very strong and reassuring, that I didn't feel too worried. I know it's strange. I've often cursed about not being more serious, more stressed about it. Well, she told me, I'm going in now. And she sounded like she was saying, Be right back.

I guess it didn't help that I came at the best of times. I caught a bus to Boston about a week and a half later, stayed in Quincy with an old friend, and spent most of only a few days with Laura, her family, and her friends. Before seeing her I saw her godmother and was introduced to two of her friends. Laura, it turned out, was recovering more rapidly than anyone had expected. When the doctors said she'd be asleep for days, she woke in hours; when we were told she'd be mute, she spoke up and joked and smiled.

She's so strong, her friends told me, it's unbelievable.

Her father came and said the same thing: She's so strong, it's unbelievable. If the nurses didn't say it outright, you could tell they were thinking it, by the way they casually came and went.

I don't remember her mother saying it, but I'm sure she thought what we all thought.

And I believe the most touching thing about the situation was that you (I) could tell she was in a good mood, and strong, for her own sake. She wasn't—as she'd done before, and as she's done since the operation has shown its flaws—looking or acting well to reassure any of us, those around her, but was elated at her own triumph and strength and stepping forward. The transplant meant so many new things for her to do . . . and Laura has often told me about her want to take on new things.

I can't help but be a sap, and say that I believe more than anything that it is Laura's own strength of will that got her through the transplant so well, that took her as far as she is today, and, most of all, carried the rest of us through it with her.

LUCY PENTLAND, MY GRANDMOTHER

I wish I could write a real account of the courageous calling of every opportunity for Laura to share the experience of a normal life, from childhood and school, right up to Laura's graduating and her acceptance at Brown University in Providence, all that time interrupted by weeks of treatment for cystic fibrosis in Presbyterian Babies' and Children's Hospital. People gathered round her to help: friends and family, hospital staff, doctors, teachers, classmates, until it was the other way round, and she was giving help to them. So this will just be a grandmother's view, from the sidelines.

After a very moving graduation of an exceptional class at Chapin, and a really wonderful party, which Laura gave for hospital staff, doctors, teachers, and everyone who had helped her to success, preparations began for moving to Providence for university life, setting up a room with all the needed electronic equipment, and the atmosphere of walls covered with photographs of her friends and family, Christmas lights to make it cheerful, and then volunteering to drive a van for campus transportation 7–11 P.M., and making contact with doctors at Rhode Island Hospital, where she gave a talk to incoming freshmen, answering as I remember questions on her attitude toward death. Several of her good friends at Presbyterian with CF had died.

When the second semester at Brown began, her coughing was getting much worse, and at one class the professor interrupted his lecture to look at her. Afterward, of course, she explained her condition to the professor. Later when there was gossip on the school computer Net about her coughing, she published an article in the school newspaper, and the professor spoke to the class about discrimination.

About this time the question became serious of getting her name listed for a transplant. After she was listed at Presbyterian Hospital in New York, the doctors there said transplants weren't successful with the type of infection she was subject to and would no longer consider her name.

The next thing I heard was that Laura had been searching the Internet on her own and had contacted a doctor at Boston Children's Hospital who did accept patients of her type. And she was going there with her father and mother for an interview. This was before Christmas 1999. A year later she was ready for the transplant.

From then on there was a time that from all sides help was gathering—from her great aunt's legacy, from her father's brother, from good friends, and the possibility of an apartment near the hospital in Boston as a home base.

Laura always needed an event to be working for—collecting for the CF walk, travel to England, Scotland, Ireland when she was able, back to New York to check in with friends, birthdays, weddings.

Eventually she was placed on the New England transplant list, and the apartments in New York and Boston were set up to have immediate contact, to go to the hospital on one hour's notice. As grandmother I wasn't really closely following each step, except that her breathing was becoming weaker or, again, a new infection and hospitalization. She had support from friends almost every weekend, even after school was out.

Eventually she was listed number one.

It was not until July, when I was in Los Angeles, quite early in the morning, that a call came through from Mary: "LAURA IS HAVING HER TRANSPLANT NOW." And there was an overwhelming surge of gratitude and tears mixed together, almost disbelief.

I have only seen photographs and heard of the actual transplant, the delivery of the donated lungs, the number of hours of surgery, the time in a coma—several days, support from all kinds of tubes, a moment of awakening but not knowing where she was, then writing, "This hospital has no fan," which was true. I remember especially a picture of her sitting up, looking beautiful, ready to go home.

Now there have followed many months of constant medical testing, procedures, changing medicines, hospitalizations. After each, it is amazing—the strength of her voice, the energy as she walks, even when she was saying the breathing was not so different than before surgery.

Of course, there has to be mentioned the care and attention of Jon and Mary, always being at hand, constantly, at every crisis, day and night.

DIANE SAWYER, FRIEND,
NEWS ANCHOR

The transplant was an education (like a crash course in medical school).

It was hope and prayer all braided into one.

It was joy, then a whiplash of worry.

Finally, feeling like a parachute opened on a free fall.

And most of all, it was Laura, full bravery, full passion, full poetry.

It was a reminder that life doesn't let us choose. But oh how it lets us love.

DIANA FISHMAN,
HIGH SCHOOL FRIEND

I went to visit Laura in Boston the spring before the transplant, when she was waiting. Since I always admired the flocks of color that floated in the corners of her rooms, Laura taught me how to fold cranes. She let me choose from her collection of subtly textured, metallic, and oriental-patterned squares, and she guided me crease by crease through the process. These same steps that at summer camp I could do with my eyes shut had no logic to me then, and I produced lopsided, crumbled cranes with no resemblance to the ones that glided gracefully across her apartment. Laura had to finish most of mine when she saw that there was no bird emerging from my knot of overcreased paper. Only a few months later, it was my fingers straightening beaks and correcting unbalanced wings.

Corner to corner, edge to edge, fold, crease, cranes bloomed out of recycled wrapping paper, shiny gum wrappers, and for the more sophisticated of us, elaborately patterned sleeves of origami paper. It became my mission, an obsession of sorts, and the only positive way I could direct my anxiety surrounding the transplant, to make 1,000 paper cranes for Laura. I am not sure whether I believed the legend—that a terminally ill person would get better if s/he received 1,000 paper cranes, or if it was just the best way I could show Laura that I loved her, that even if I could not be with her, I thought about her all the time.

During camp free times, when I saw an idle camper, aimlessly wondering or staring at nothing at all, lost in the imagination of adolescence, I sat down next to him or her and asked, "Do you know how to make cranes? Do you want to learn?" And so the mission continued. Each day I counted and recorded the mounting number as the crane box became a little more full. Each day, I strung cranes together on clear wire, alternating colors and sizes and balancing the number of awkwardly folded mishaps to perfectly creased cranes.

But when the day came, the cranes were not finished. Not only were there not 1,000 paper cranes, but I wasn't even at camp, I was still asleep in my boyfriend's house in New York when my mother's call came. The cell phone did not serve its original purpose. When I woke up to the news that Laura was under and getting new lungs, I felt somehow betrayed that I wasn't woken up when the news first came, and distressed that at the crucial moment I wasn't closer to Boston. I had just seen Laura a week or two before in her apartment in Boston with some friends. We ate and tried to laugh and talk. She looked as gorgeous and spunky as ever, even with the clear tube flowing oxygen into her nostrils, easing her tired breath. She had stopped doing a lot of activity, and life had become waiting.

On the Sunday morning in July when the call came, I did not want to believe that my last visit may have been *the last* visit. Yet that possibility hovered over my head, like the less-than 1,000 paper cranes that hung from the art studio walls at my summer camp. We deliberated over whether to go immediately to sit with the others in the hospital waiting room, or to worry on our own. We decided that Laura's parents had people with them, and the type of support they needed was out of our capacity to give. So the cell phone went back into use for updates.

About a week after the surgery, a week of hearing from afar about the tremors and pain Laura was experiencing, a week of factory-style crane production, my boyfriend and I went to Boston to see Laura. We were two of the first friends to get to see her. I brought a bouquet of tissue paper flowers made by my campers because she could not have any real flowers in her immune-suppressed state. I didn't know what to say, and I felt myself gawking, overwhelmed with awe. Laura showed us the digital photographs of her old, shriveled, blackened lungs and the new, fleshy, healthy ones. She was excited, proud, though still struggling with the reality of post-transplant life. Time in the sterile room stood still, and yet I never wanted to leave, just in case—but Laura kept fighting, as she always has for the seven or eight years that I've known her.

I was going to spend the next semester in Niger, West Africa, with no phone, certainly no cell phone for daily updates. In the midst of mind-racing packing and preparation to go somewhere I couldn't comprehend, Laura stopped at my apartment to say good-bye on her way up to Providence. I picked up my oversized box of cranes and headed downstairs to deliver them. There weren't quite 1,000, though we were close, perhaps nine hundred something. And after weeks of crazed paper cutting and folding and stringing, I realized the number didn't so much matter. The cranes, unlike the cell phone, served their purpose. As we hugged good-bye, tears formed films in our eyes, I knew that it was more than worth the effort. Laura understood how much I loved her.

RUTH ROTHENBERG, MY NANA, DICTATES ————————

Writes Aunt Judy: I did get it together this afternoon to ask Nana about her reactions to the transplant. Here's what she said:

1) The transplant caused a whole lot of worry for everyone.

2) Her hopes for the transplant were that you would have a whole new life.

3) The transplant kept everyone in the family in close contact with one another.

4) The transplant made her appreciate each day she had a normal day's life.

5) The transplant helped her decide to make the decision to come to California. She figured if you were "going to take the plunge," a big plunge at that, then she could do it, too.

JANE L. RINDEN, HIGH SCHOOL
ENGLISH TEACHER ————————————

In the Seraglio

Like Scheherazade, she nightly weaves her stories,
out to outwit fate.
They fly to us as e-mail,
fueled with medical terms we've never heard,
the heroine always caught in a quandary with
no way out;
the action set mainly in the Northeast corridor,
in out-of-the-way apartments, hospital rooms,
or racing cars.
Drama builds to the climax
and we hold our breath,
next sequence simmering into tomorrow.
She is the master of our emotions,
manipulating heartstrings,
while we root for her release.

CHRISTOPHER SALES,
COLLEGE FRIEND ————————————

I remember feeling nervous that you would die before you
had the transplant. When Diana and Josh and I came to visit
you that weekend before your transplant I was worried that you

wouldn't get the new lungs in time. I could see you getting weaker. But at the same time, I was also scared about the transplant itself. I didn't know if you would make it through the procedure; what if you died?

So I brought my camera. I told myself; these pictures are for Laura and all of those people who love and care about Laura, especially her parents. If she doesn't get the lungs, or if the transplant doesn't work out, I want Laura and her loved ones to have these pictures.

I remember making a decision the weekend before the transplant to sacrifice spending time with you just so that I could take photos *for* you. In fact, my girlfriend and I had an argument (afterward) about me being detached from the social atmosphere when we visited; she thought I was being selfish by being caught up in my photography. I explained how I felt like my photos were not for myself, but for you and your parents. Anyway, so as you probably recall, I took an enormous number of photos that day. And every time that I clicked the shutter, I felt like I was running out of time. What if the last photo that I took was not good? So I would take another and another just in case . . . just in case you died. And that was really how I felt.

In the time after your transplant, as you gradually recovered . . . I decided to forgo the photographic "duty." I began to feel like much of the time that I spent with you was done proximately through a lens. So I put down my camera, and since then, I have not really picked it up much. Instead I've tried (with not much success) to just spend time with you. And amid the days of busy-ness that pass, I wonder why I haven't.

MRS. PUTNAM, HIGH SCHOOL
ENGLISH TEACHER

My first memories of Laura at Chapin coincided with first learning about CF through another student, who died as a senior. Her wrenching coughs were echoed by those of a much younger child, Laura. Both had devoted classmates who were so frustrated by the power of the disease that they fund-raised their hearts out to contribute to research. The CF walk every year gave everyone, students and teachers, a chance to join the fight in honor of Amanda and Laura. Laura was a fine, sensitive, enthusiastic English student. She had to miss a lot of class, and I missed her so much that I used to go up to Columbia Presbyterian to visit with her. That room—all those hospital rooms through the years—testimonies to the love of her friends, to the enduring energy and engagement of Laura's family, and to the girl Laura. Very much a girl, she had to be really, really sick not to notice if a resident was cut or if he had paid appropriate attention to her! Laura had made close friends in all those hospital visits.

Odd word, visits: sometimes it seemed she was more in the hospital than at home. I do remember how much Laura became part of the hospital community. For one thing, she was really interested in other patients, and she was a spark for the ones who needed it. I often thought she was part of what kept the nurses going, too. (Whether it was at Presbyterian or later in Boston at Children's, I was proud to tell them who my friend was—the nurses always brightened up, especially if there was good news at the time.) Her friends would get their hopes up that she was getting better and would come out soon, and then despair if she had a relapse. A lot of our life at Chapin was preoccupied with Laura—what was her phone number this time, did she feel like talking, how was she reacting to the medication, to the latest bronch, to the loss of one of her CF friends?

Getting our hopes up—that was a lot of the seesaw or roller coaster that was Laura's CF. She would come back and star in a dressed-up, sophisticated role in a play, and then, bang, back into the hospital. Or she would organize a birthday celebration for one of her friends, and she'd be back in the hospital. The rest of us would droop, but we were only on the sidelines. I remember the day she turned eighteen, and there was a big cake for her classmates, but soon Laura took some time out in a conference room, aware of the knife-edge irony that she felt "middle-aged," particularly having just lost another friend to CF.

When the possibility of transplant came, Laura was absolutely ready to put herself forward. Those ensuing months of waiting and not knowing were long, very long for someone like Laura who wants to make things happen. For her friends, she rallied in letters, phone calls, and visiting about. My husband and I were reassured when she cheerfully came over to have breakfast or tea when we visited in Boston. No matter what was going on with her, before and after the transplant, Laura was open and patient about teaching us what was going on and what her options were. I often wondered how she could be so much fun in those days. I hoped it didn't cost her too much to be that way with so very many friends.

The transplant itself was a miraculous event covered like the walk on the moon by her friends who were on the spot. The phone calls and the e-mails were beautiful and detailed and established an extraordinary network of friends who cared deeply about the success of that operation. I'm sorry I wasn't on hand, but I felt as if I were. EB's reporting was Pulitzer Prize stuff. Our first actual visit after the operation was joyous. (It was also before some of the complications.) The staff was cautiously jubilant, just so happy for this young person they had come to value. As usual, we had to suit up, but it felt well worth it. Also as usual, her room was a shrine to her friends and family, with photos and cards and posters, balloons, animals everywhere. No flowers, I think, still. Her friend from New Hampshire had come down to see her, and they were plotting mischief already.

One thing I remember through this time was Laura's persistent support of a schoolmate down in New York who had suddenly come down with leukemia. Laura called her often—not many other youngsters know firsthand about life-threatening diseases. Laura also called an old resident friend from Presbyterian days and made sure he visited K. in New York Hospital. That old loyalty for a former schoolmate was a lovely thing for their former teacher to see.

Through her school years, Laura had her abiding passion for writing. She did not write only about CF, but as the disease closed in, she wrote and she wrote. Through her writing, we grew to understand more about other patients and about the doctors. Laura wrote stories, plays, poems, and nonfiction reminiscences. Laura was brave, inventive, and shrewd in her writing. She provided remarkable insights for her readers. It was a lifeline for her, and she wanted to do it as well as possible. She was trying to understand why this was happening to her and what she could do about it. She was almost clinically interested in the ways others perceived her. And she was determined not to be defined by the disease. There is no question that she broke the mold.

JANE SEIDES, MY AUNT

I hoped, dreamed, and prayed that Laura would get a new set of lungs and with them, a better chance in life. We learned that she was having her transplant a few hours before our thirty-fifth wedding anniversary. We cried, prayed, worried, and laughed all at the same time. Laura's new chance was the most precious, poignant gift we could ever have received to celebrate that day. I felt God's presence and blessing, for her and for us.

STEVE LEVIN, COLLEGE FRIEND

There are critical times in life. Situations that only existed in our minds become physical and so powerful that they eclipse all other aspects of life. This could be found in a person's search for love, a runaway train, or a soldier's battle. Usually, there is something a person can do, a decision one can make, an action one can take that could influence or, at times, totally dictate the critical outcome. This gives us a sense of power and confidence that is false.

The element of coincidence and chance is totally beyond us and, I suppose, this is what we call faith. We also call it hope, whether that hope lives through God, love, suffering, or joy. In the face of the most incredible and trying times, the critical times, hope and faith are essential for us to understand who we are. I am certain Laura Rothenberg knows this well. She has helped teach it to me.

CAROL DEBOER-LANGWORTHY, ENGLISH PROFESSOR AT BROWN UNIVERSITY

In spring 2000, I offered "Lifewriting" for the second time as an expository writing course at Brown University. This was still a fairly new course and I was looking for teaching strategies. Someone suggested a neat idea: have the kids write their obituaries! It would elicit their expectations of the rest of their lives, and help them to reflect on their lives thus far as well.

So I made this the first assignment. Two days later, before the students handed in their writing, I asked the class members to go around the table and read their opening paragraphs. Most of the students had written of themselves dying at around age eighty. By that time they had at least two professional degrees beyond college, had traveled the world, were successful in love and family life, and were leaving at least one book behind from their sojourn on earth.

Then we came to Laura. I don't have a copy of what she wrote, but its substance sticks in the mind. She began by saying that she had a different standard for success. She didn't know what the next three months would bring, much less the next four years. But she was living her life as though there were a happy ending, and that each moment was a treasure. She told us about cystic fibrosis and expressed her long-term prognosis in medical terms. I don't recall whether she said the word *transplant* or not. But she did talk about writing and how happy she was to be sitting at this table at this time. All this she conveyed calmly, with her clear-eyed courage.

We were stunned and I was chagrined. (This is no longer the opening assignment for this course.) Immediately, our class discussions became far more nuanced and less glossy. We all felt permission to reveal our doubts, fears, and regrets—which probably would not have been the case so early in the course without Laura's bold lead. Thus was my initiation to the world of CF and to following Laura's journey as detailed on these pages. It has been a fascinating ride, even though I'm not altogether proud of my performance.

Needless to say, Laura's presence in the classroom enriched us. We bonded and always looked forward to Laura's "take" on any given assignment. A famous incident was her discussion of veins for another early assignment, the so-called body piece. Working in small groups, students read their work aloud to each other. I wandered around Horace Mann Hall, the old English Department building full of nooks and crannies, listening in on gaggles of lifewriters reading to each other. Rounding a corner to a student lounge, I noted Mollie L. dizzily groping her way along the wall to the women's bathroom. Turns out Mollie, a tough premedical student with nerves of steel, had been nearly undone by Laura's eloquent description of her circulatory system. Powerful writing!

LATOYA SUTTON, HIGH SCHOOL FRIEND

It's hard to explain Laura to other people. She's more than the average twenty-one-year-old, but I hate to define her by an illness. I try to tell my friends who did not go to high school with me about the amazing person I am friends with, and I never feel like I am doing her justice. It makes it hard to express my feelings about her because I feel like I am part of this special club that knows this wonderful person and has a different better life because of this, but most people don't have a clue what it's like. When I first learned that she was going to go on the transplant list I thought that I was okay, that I could handle it just like any other event in the past years. When she told me she was leaving school to move to Boston and wait for new lungs, once again I thought I was okay. One day after hearing her speak about cystic fibrosis to a group of first-year med students, I walked to lunch at the Ratty . . . and promptly burst out crying when my friends asked me how her lecture was.

The day I got the call that the transplant was under way, I was shopping for school supplies in Target. I clearly remember being in the juice aisle when my phone rang. I didn't know whether to laugh, cry, or faint. Honestly I wanted to tell everyone in the store, "EVERYONE PAY ATTENTION, THIS IS BIG. SOMETHING INCREDIBLE IS HAPPENING!!" How can you shop for socks when my friend is undergoing a life changing surgery? I explained to my mom what was happening while I called my best friend to keep the telephone chain alive. For the rest of the day I felt completely helpless, wishing to be in Boston, but knowing that it was an impossibility. Instead, I called for updates from her roommate and tried to keep my blood pressure down.

I walked into Laura's apartment in New York in August of 2001, a few weeks after her transplant. I remembered the first time that I walked into her apartment, for a costumed birthday party in eighth grade. I was still getting used to my new school, but even then I knew that I had found a friend in Laura. But this past August, I was amazed by the fact that just a few years before I had associated Laura's house with themed birthday parties and sleepovers, and now it was here for a completely different kind of celebration.

In the fall of 2001 I spent the semester abroad in Barbados. I had limited e-mail capabilities but I always waited anxiously for Laura's update e-mails. I was feeling a bit detached from the United States and it frustrated me no end. Though I looked for them, it was always difficult for me to read her e-mails because of all the medical jargon that went along with describing the latest infection or complication with the transplant. Though Laura did her best to explain it, I was pretty confused most of the time. I was always left with the question: "But are you okay?" For the first time since I had known her I wasn't able to go and visit her and see her with my own eyes. I couldn't look into her eyes and see that unmistakable Laura, and it scared the heck out of me. Sometimes after reading an e-mail I would end up crying while my boyfriend tried to comfort me, confused because I couldn't explain the entire story to him.

My parents ask about Laura often, knowing how important she is to me. Over Christmas break my father commented (imagine this spoken in a West Indian accent): "That Laura is special. She's a real survivor." I agree with him. Knowing Laura is like riding a roller coaster. It's a little scary and pretty fast-paced but it also takes you to amazing heights and incredible thrills. I am a better person for having the luck to have her in my life. I wouldn't trade her friendship for anything.

MEGAN NICOLAY,
FORMER BROWN STUDENT ———————————

Because She Breathes for a Living

a frame, fitted to her shoulders
built to carry

a load in two equal portions:

lungs yoked
the words spoken,
choked on
for the time being
she waits for a new machine

I remember that poetry (of machines)
and she, waiting for a new one
a new poem; a new machine

to be healed by knives, branded
a smile carved into her chest—
she too breathes for a living
this is my bad lung, she says
it sits in a dish (at the bedside).

with stories of mucus
and clotted breath.

she knows the tangles intimately. the wires, like
   arms and legs.
the tubes run from her body like escaping veins.
the scars, an exotic necklace clinging to her chest.

getting whole again
she's breathing and
doesn't even notice

we got the word and it was like
she
spoke it twice
for quiet emphasis
she spoke it twice
to prove it was really there—

          *   *   *

I do not know which to prefer,
   The beauty of inflections
Or the beauty of innuendoes,
   The blackbird whistling
     Or just after.
—Wallace Stevens

Epilogue

JANUARY 9, 2003 —————————————————————

So first I was crazy. But we fixed that with medication. Then, last summer, as the result of an unfortunate roller-blading accident on the sidewalk corner of 71st and Second, I broke my hip. Had surgery for it. I managed to make it to the wedding of a dear friend in Atlanta, just as I received the last drop of a four-unit blood transfusion and returned to New York City to start my summer internship at the Legal Aid Society, only a week late.

My transplant anniversary rolled around a few weeks thereafter, and I was quite skeptical about my second year, seeing as my last biopsy had shown acute rejection. The doctors reassured me that it didn't mean anything. As always, I had a premonition of what was to come and, as always, I was right.

The fall of 2002 consisted of a series of hospitalizations on 8 North, during which I reconnected with some of my favorite younger transplant patients, not to mention the nurses and other staff. And at a certain point, I just stopped leaving the hospital. However, I did make it out for two trips, one to New York City and one to Maine with Bryan, my boyfriend.

It was advanced medicine, more so than it had been the first year, to the point where most general practitioners wouldn't understand the intricacies of my case. Certain radiologists had to read my films, certain surgeons had to perform my surgeries. More bronchs, more biopsies, more questions, and by Thanksgiving I was moving back to New York because I was diagnosed with chronic rejection and there was no longer anything curative that could be done.

I think I found an apartment in the fastest time possible for a New Yorker looking in Manhattan. Bryan and I moved in together, but I wasn't able to go to Virginia at Christmastime to see his family. I was simply too sick. Instead, I spent what will probably be my last Christmas, not at home with my parents, but in the hospital. In my long history of hospitalizations, it was the only holiday that I had not previously spent in the hospital.

I left the hospital on New Year's Eve on more oxygen than ever before. Went straight to the hairdresser and then back to my new apartment to get ready for the evening that was planned. Bryan and I barely made it to our own party because of how slow I had become. Around 150 people were waiting on the boat that we had rented; many were friends, many others were friends by association. We made it as close as we could to the Statue of Liberty at midnight and while watching the fireworks I was surrounded by four of the most important people in my life.

Tonight, in the PICU at Mt. Sinai I watched a baby get intubated across the hall. As usual, the nurse came into my room saying, "Sorry I'm late, we had an emergency," as if I didn't have the eyes to see what was happening myself. A long time ago I stopped counting how many of my friends in the hospital had died, how many other children had died, but I do remember how scared my friend Sophie looked when she was dying at age seventeen. Her eyes pierced through the glass window at Columbia Hospital. Even though she was delirious, she saw me, she waved, and fell back into her delirium.

And now I'm aware of my short-term memory loss, my increased need for oxygen, my moments where I struggle with the question of whether it's easier to live or to die. In the end, I come to the conclusion that I want to live, but . . . How can I resign myself to death if my biggest fear is not being able to breathe?

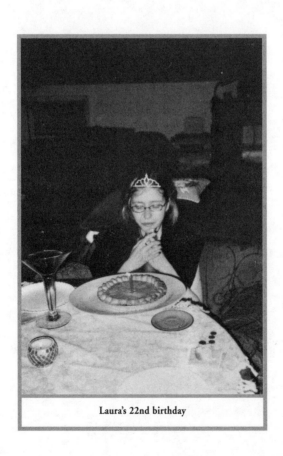

Laura's 22nd birthday